Aesthetics for the Therapist

Also published by Stanley Thornes (Publishers) Ltd:

W E Arnould-Taylor	*The Principles and Practice of Physical Therapy*
Ann Gallant	*Body Treatments and Dietetics for the Beauty Therapist*
Ann Gallant	*Principles and Techniques for the Beauty Specialist*
Ann Gallant	*Principles and Techniques for the Electrologist*
John Rounce	*Science for the Beauty Therapist*

Please write to the publishers for further details.

Aesthetics for the Therapist

Ann Hagman SRN, Cert Ed, DAES, MPhys

Stanley Thornes (Publishers) Ltd

First published in 1991 by:
Stanley Thornes (Publishers) Ltd

Reprinted in 2002 by:
Nelson Thornes Ltd
Delta Place
27 Bath Road
CHELTENHAM
GL53 7TH
United Kingdom

02 03 04 05 / 15 14 13 12 11

A catalogue record for this book is available from the British Library

ISBN 0 7487 0566 X

Page make-up by Tech-Set, Gateshead, Tyne and Wear

Printed and bound in Great Britain by Scotprint

This book is dedicated to all former tutors and students of Wendover House College
from whom I have learnt so much, and to my husband Ronald Hagman
for his loyal support and understanding.

Contents

Foreword

In his foreword to Ann Hagman's original text book *The Aestheticienne, simple theory and practice* published in 1981, William Arnould-Taylor, Chairman of the International Therapy Examination Council wrote:

'It gives me much pleasure to write a foreword for a book which was specially commissioned for ITEC but which will obviously fill the much greater need of an easily understandable textbook for general Aestheticienne education.

The author, Ann Hagman, is very well qualified to write such a book. As a State Registered Nurse of considerable experience she has a wide knowledge of people and their needs. To this experience is added that of being Principal of a private Beauty Therapy training school as well as running a successful clinic – a happy combination of theory and practice.

In wishing the book all the success which I am sure it will achieve I would commend it to all schools and colleges undertaking any aspect of Beautician/Aestheticienne training'.

Ten years later I am delighted to write the foreword for a most worthy successor to *The Aestheticienne*. *Aesthetics for the Therapist* is the culmination of months of dedicated work by Ann Hagman. The experience she has gained during the intervening ten years in the much broader range of therapies which come under the group heading of 'aesthetics' has been expertly committed to paper. Students are indeed fortunate to have this knowledge at their fingertips.

The text has been laid out in a completely new format which facilitates study, and the new illustrations complement the work to provide a clear, concise and readable book for anyone who is interested in the fascinating subject of 'beauty'.

Kim Aldridge
Director General
The International Therapy Examination Council
Limited
1991

Preface

Writing a textbook can be rather like a pregnancy. First there is a long gestation period when all the ideas for the text and artwork are put down on paper and checked for details and accuracy. Then the rush when proof-reading and indexing must take place immediately prior to printing. It is very exciting to hold the first copy; to examine the cover and look at the diagrams and type of print. Then the book must leave 'home' to help others to work.

This book is written for students all over the world who are going to take a beauty course. In several instances different methods of performing a treatment have been included. Tutors and other therapists will no doubt have their own ideas. There are many ways of performing even such a simple treatment as a manicure. Just because it is not the same as the way that you are used to performing it does not mean that it is wrong. It is just different. Do not criticise others just because they perform differently from you, but instead perhaps, be prepared to learn new methods.

Beauty is still a mainly female orientated career. The female gender has been used throughout the text. I apologise to any man who might feel slighted on this account. It was done for speed of writing as much as for semantics and rhythm of reading.

Ann Hagman
1991

Acknowledgements

The writer wishes to thank personally the following people and organisations for their assistance in producing this book.

Ms. Francis Alright, The Association of Sun Tanning Operators, London; for information on ultraviolet. Mrs. Christine Campbell-Salisbury, Marbella Hair and Beauty College, Marbella, Spain; for details of the Spanish treatment. Ms. Lindsey Cole, Southgate, London; for general content reading and advice. Mrs. Marie Faux-Jones, West of England College, Bath, England and Tokyo, Japan; for details of the Japanese massage. Mrs. Shahnaz Husain, Nilofar School, New Delhi, India; for information on eye care. Mr. Don Jackson and Mr. David Pewsey, Hospital Equipment Laboratory Products Ltd, London; for technical details. Longman Group UK for reproduction of extracts from *Harry's Cosmeticology*, ed. Wilkinson and Moore. Ms. Vanessa Puttick, The Hairdressing & Beauty Equipment Centre, London; for technical details. The Director and staff of Ronald Hagman Ltd, London; for technical details. Mrs. Vera Roper, Afrodite School, Nairobi, Kenya for details of the African facial. The Editorial Directors and artistic designers, Stanley Thornes, Cheltenham; for advice and artwork. The members of The International Therapy Examination Council, England; for advice and support.

PART A

Anatomy and Physiology

Chapter I

Introduction

Today, everybody wants to look good as well as to feel good. The aestheticienne or body therapist is someone who can help to achieve this.

In order to perform treatments upon clients, the therapist should have a clear understanding of what goes on in the body. Thus a good knowledge of anatomy and physiology is essential.

To make learning easier, the anatomy section has been divided into eight parts: the six main systems, the skin and the accessory organs (hands, feet, nails, hair and breasts). No system should be viewed in total isolation as no system can function on its own, but always works in conjunction with others. As the therapist works over a specific area she must be aware that a number of systems may be affected by her work.

Basic Terminology

The therapist should have some knowledge of the basic terminology used.

Anatomy The study of the structure of the body.
Physiology The study of the functions of the systems of the body.
Histology The microscopic study of tissue.
Pathology The study of a disease.
Morphology The study of structure and form.
Natural anatomical position The human body in an erect position, with the arms hanging loosely by the side and the palms of the hand facing forward.
Anterior or **ventral view** The front aspect of the body in the erect position.
Posterior or **dorsal view** The rear aspect of the body in the erect position.
Median line The vertical central line of a structure, e.g. an imaginary line running through the centre of the body from the crown of the head to between the feet.
Medial Towards the median line of the body, e.g. the inner side of the arm.
Lateral Furthest away from the median line, e.g. the outer side of the arm.

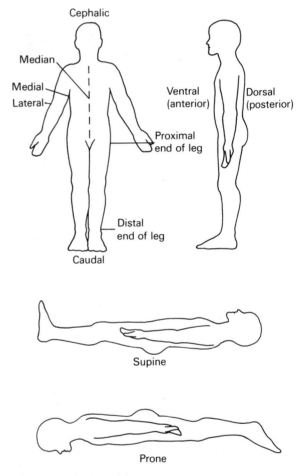

The anatomical positions

Proximal Nearest to the heart or median line, e.g. the hip is at the 'proximal' end of the leg.
Distal Furthest away from the heart or median line, e.g. the ankle is at the 'distal' end of the leg.
Peripheral The surface or outer edge, e.g. the skin is 'peripheral' to the rest of the body.
Superficial Lying nearest the surface, e.g. the epidermis is the most 'superficial' layer of the skin.
Deep Away from the surface, e.g. the heart lies 'deep' within the thorax.

Symmetrical When both sides of the body are similar or in harmony, e.g. both ears are at the same height.

Superior or **cephalic** Towards the head and upper part of the body.

Inferior or **caudal** Away from the head, towards the lower part of the body.

Supine In the horizontal position, lying on the back.

Prone In the horizontal position, lying face downwards.

Afferent Towards.

Efferent Away from.

Chapter 2

Cells, Tissues, Metabolism and the Immune System

CELLS

All living matter is made up of *cells*. They are the smallest single units of life. They vary in size, shape, structure and function.

In humans, the first single cell (*zygote*) is produced by the fusion of the female egg (*ovum*) and the male cell (*spermatozoon*).

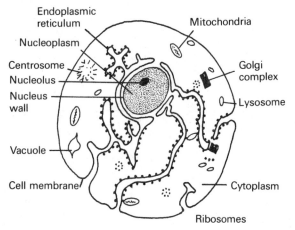

Endoplasmic reticulum
Mitochondria
Nucleoplasm
Centrosome
Nucleolus
Golgi complex
Nucleus wall
Lysosome
Vacuole
Cell membrane
Cytoplasm
Ribosomes

A cell

Cell Structure

Surrounding each cell is a very fine membrane. This is semi-permeable, having pores. These allow certain substances to enter and leave the cell by one of four methods:

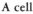

diffusion
osmosis
phagocytosis
active transport.

Diffusion

The substances may be a liquid such as water, or a gas such as oxygen or carbon dioxide. These may be diffused by the higher concentration passing through the membrane to the lower concentration.

Osmosis

Here water is drawn through the membranes from the weaker solution to the stronger.

Phagocytosis

Liquids or particles such as fatty lipids may be engulfed by the membrane and then dissolved before passing into the cell.

Active Transport

Substances such as glucose and amino acids are linked to specific carriers in the cell wall. They are then transported through the cell wall and released.

All human cells contain a mass called *protoplasm* which resembles the white of an egg. This forms the *cytoplasm* or body of the cell. It consists of protein, carbohydrates, water, lipids and electrolytes. *Nucleoplasm* is a similar substance. This is encased by the nuclear membrane within a section of the cell called the nucleus.

The Nucleus

The nucleus is the centre of activity for the cell. It contains a special type of protein (*nucleoprotein*) that controls the chemical reaction within the cell and also the reproduction of that cell. There are a number of thread-like processes in the nucleus called *chromosomes*. They appear as a dark, stained mass called *chromatin*.

Each chromosome thread consists of a number of smaller chains which resemble beads. These are called *genes*. Genes are made from long strands of *deoxyribonucleic acid* (DNA). This in turn is made up of four different molecules collectively called *nucleotides*. These link together to form a *double helix* rather like a spiralling ladder. On one side are sugars and phosphates. On the other side can be any one of four different base compounds.

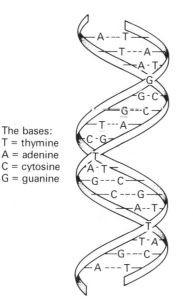

The bases:
T = thymine
A = adenine
C = cytosine
G = guanine

A double helix

Genes carry and pass on all the hereditary information of the parents. This includes information on the colour of the eyes, hair and skin, and also on blood groups, certain hereditary diseases and congenital defects.

Genes may be referred to as *dominant* when they have a strong influence, or *recessive* when their effectiveness is reduced.

Both the ovum and spermatozoon carry 23 chromosomes. When these join together to form the *zygote*, this has 23 chromosomes from each parent; 46 chromosomes in all.

The sex of a person depends on the sex chromosomes. The female has a pair of X chromosomes (XX). The male has mixed chromosomes (XY). The sex of the baby is determined by whether it inherited the X or the Y chromosome from the father.

The Organelles

Within the cytoplasm or body of the cell lie a number of other structures. They are called *organelles*. They include:

Ribosomes

DNA is capable of reproducing itself and of stimulating the ribosomes through the formation of *ribonucleic acid* (RNA). This transmits genetic information to the cells' protein for synthesis in the cell.

Endoplasmic Reticulum

This is a fine network of tubules which connects the nucleus to the cell membrane. Substances are transported from one part of the cell to another through the tubules. Ribosomes line the endoplasmic reticulum, but can also be found on other surfaces within the cells.

Mitochondria

These are very small structures which extract energy from nutrients and oxygen. This is then stored as *adenosine triphosphate* (ATP) and is later used for cellular activities.

Lysosomes

These are small structures which remove and digest unwanted particles in the cell through the action of enzymes.

Vacuoles

These are clear spaces where waste matter may be kept prior to secretion from the cell.

Golgi Bodies

These are the structures that secrete the waste matter from the cells.

Centrosomes

These are made up of two small, round bodies called *centrioles*. They play a major part in cell division.

Life Cycle of a Cell

New cells are continually required by the body throughout its life. They are first needed for the growth of each organ and then to replace the worn-out cells. When a body is growing, cells are reproduced at a rapid rate. Some cells, such as those in the bone marrow (where blood cells are produced) will continue the rapid reproduction process throughout life. Others, such as muscle cells, reproduce at a slower rate. Certain nerve cells are unable to reproduce at all when damaged.

Cell Reproduction: Mitosis

The manner in which cells reproduce themselves is called *mitosis*. There are four main stages:

prophase
metaphase
anaphase
telophase.

Prophase

The parent cell starts the process of dividing into two daughter cells. The centrosome divides into two centrioles. These migrate to opposite ends of the cell but remain joined by fine spindle threads. The chromatin material alters into well-defined chromosomes. These divide into two complete sets but remain joined by a strand called a *centromere*.

Metaphase

The nuclear membrane fragments and then disperses. The chromosomes arrange themselves at the centre of the nucleus and attach themselves to the spindle threads.

Anaphase

The centromere stretches as the centrioles are drawn further apart. The chromosomes then split and move towards the end of the cell. The fine spindle threads of the centrioles then divide to form new centrosomes.

Telophase

A new nuclear membrane forms around each set of chromosomes. The spindle threads disappear. The cell membrane and the cytoplasm alter shape causing a constriction between the two new nuclei. Finally the old parent cell divides into two new identical cells. The chromosomes change to become the thread-like chromatin.

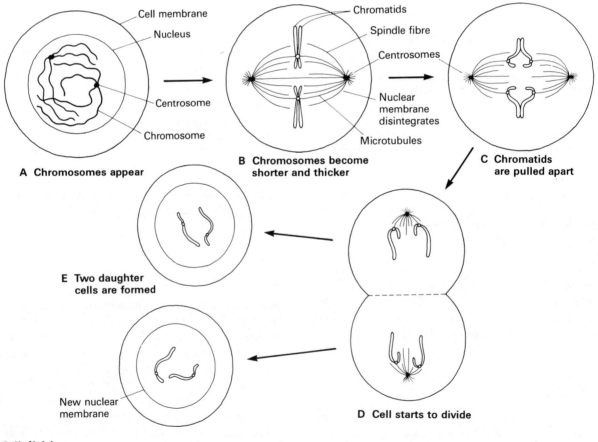

A Chromosomes appear

Cell membrane
Nucleus
Centrosome
Chromosome

B Chromosomes become shorter and thicker

Chromatids
Spindle fibre
Centrosomes
Nuclear membrane disintegrates
Microtubules

C Chromatids are pulled apart

D Cell starts to divide

E Two daughter cells are formed

New nuclear membrane

Cell division

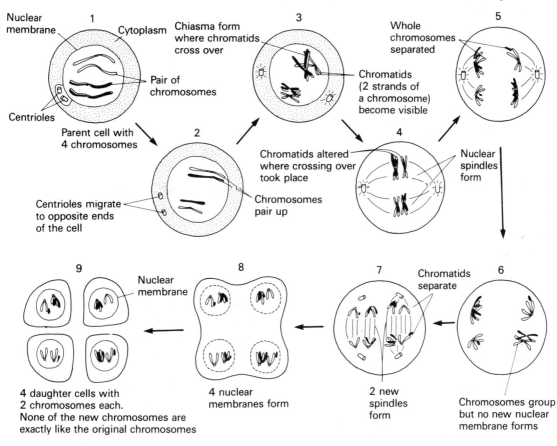

Stages in meiosis

Cell Reproduction: Meiosis

This is another form of cell division. When the *gametes* (ovum and spermatozoon) are divided they each have only half of the genetic information. It is only when the ovum is joined by the spermatozoon that there is a complete set of 46 chromosomes.

TISSUES

Tissue is formed from a collection of cells having a similar structure and function. Tissues differ in appearance according to type and function. There are four main tissue types. They are:

    epithelial tissue
    connective tissue
    muscular tissue
    nervous tissue.

Tissue Fluid

Fluid circulates around the body in several forms. When it is found inside the cells it is called *intracellular fluid*. Fluid found outside the cells is called *extracellular fluid*. This includes the fluid found in the spaces between the cells, which exchanges with blood plasma through the capillary walls. The purpose of this fluid is to transport food and oxygen from the arterial blood to the cells and return waste matter to the venous system.

Epithelial Tissue

There are several different kinds of epithelial tissue. They may be classified into two types: *simple epithelial tissue* and *compound epithelial tissue*.

Simple Epithelial Tissue

This is usually found as a single layer lying on a base membrane. Simple epithelial tissue may be subdivided according to the shape of the cells that make it up. The shape differs according to function. There are four types of simple epithelial cells:

    squamous cells
    columnar cells
    ciliated cells
    transitional cells.

Squamous Epithelial Tissue

This may also be called *pavement epithelial tissue*. The cells form a single interlocking layer that is flattened rather like a pavement. It forms a thin, smooth lining sometimes called *epithelium*. It is found in the lining of the heart, the blood and lymph vessels and the alveoli of the lungs.

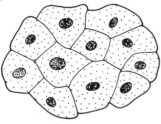

Squamous epithelial tissue

Columnar Epithelial Tissue
This is a single layer of cylindrical cells lying closely together. It is found lining the stomach and the alimentary tract. Some of the cells absorb digested food and fluids while others secrete a protective fluid called *mucus*.

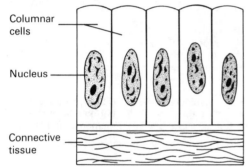

Columnar epithelial tissue

Ciliated Epithelial Tissue
This is made up of cells similar to those in columnar epithelial tissue but with the addition of fine, hair-like protrusions called *cilia*. The purpose of the cilia is to perform a sweeping type of movement in one direction. The action will convey dust, mucus or foreign bodies from the lungs, bronchi, and trachea to the throat; or clear the nasal cavities to the exterior surface. These cells are also found lining the fallopian tubes. Here their function is to propel the ovum towards the uterus.

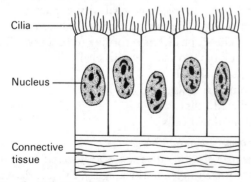

Ciliated epithelial tissue

Transitional Epithelial Tissue
This is sometimes referred to as *cuboidal epithelial tissue*. The cells lie like a single layer of cubes. They are capable of expanding and so provide a watertight surface. They are found lining the urinary tract and also the excretory glands such as the salivary glands and the breasts.

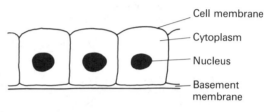

Transitional epithelial tissue

Compound Epithelial Tissue
This consists of a number of layers of cells. They grow from below and are shed when they reach the surface. They may lie on top of other layers of epithelial tissue. There are two main types:
  stratified epithelial tissue
  transitional epithelial tissue.

Compound Stratified Epithelial Tissue
This is subdivided into two categories:

a) Non-Keratinised Stratified Epithelial Tissue
These layers are specially adapted to protect under-lying tissue from wear and tear. The lower, new layers may be round in shape but become flatter as they grow nearer to the surface. They may be found in the lining of the mouth, pharynx and oesophagus, and the conjunctiva of the eye.

b) Keratinised Stratified Epithelial Tissue
These are dry, horny flattened cells containing *keratin*. They prevent the cells below from drying out. They are found on the surface of the skin, the hair and nails.

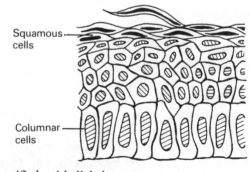

Stratified epithelial tissue

Compound Transitional Epithelial Tissue
Like the simple transitional epithelial tissue, this forms a watertight layer. It is formed from several layers of pear-shaped cells. It gives added protection to the urinary tract and vagina.

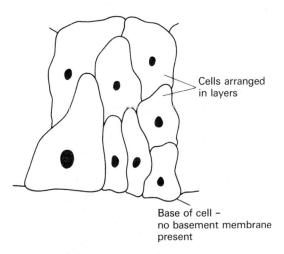

Compound transitional epithelial tissue

Connective Tissue

Connective tissue (*areolar tissue*) consists of a semi-solid ground substance called a *matrix*. This has extra-cellular fibres and cells interspersed within it.

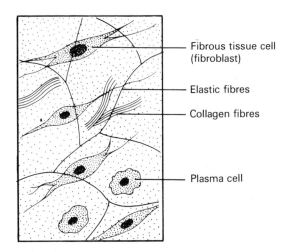

Areolar tissue

Connective tissue is the most abundant form of tissue found in the body. There are more differences found in connective tissues than in other tissues. They range from the jelly-like substance found inside

the eye (vitreous humour) to the very hard substance called bone. The differences are, however, divided into just two main categories: *loose connective tissue* and *dense connective tissue*.

Sometimes a third type may be called *fascial tissue*. The cells of connective tissue are not as closely packed together as in epithelial tissue.

Connective tissue is found in most parts of the body. It is sometimes called supportive tissue because it connects and supports other tissue such as the skin, muscles, blood vessels, nerves, alimentary tract and secretory glands.

Loose Connective Tissue
The matrix consists of protein in the form of *mucopolysaccharides*. These form a gel which is kept in a stable condition by the action of an enzyme called *hyaluronidase*. The mucopolysaccharides are ionised, and can therefore carry free negative charges. By this means certain substances can be carried around the body.

Extra-Cellular Tissue
In loose connective tissue there are two types of extracellular tissue:
a) *collagen* (known as white fibrous tissue)
b) *elastin* (known as yellow elastic tissue).

a) Collagen Fibres
These do not stretch or branch and are arranged in bundles which have a wavy appearance. They have a few cells interspersed through the fibrous bundles. The smallest collagen fibres are called *reticular fibres*. They are most numerous in embryonic tissue. In adults they are found as a network of tissue surrounding the blood and lymph vessels, nerves, muscles and bone tissue.

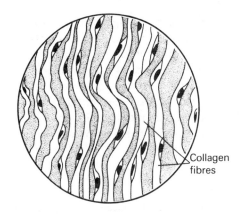

Collagen fibres

b) Elastin Fibres

These are almost the opposite of collagen. Elastin fibres have branches which can form into web-like structures. They can also stretch and then return to their original shape. They decrease in number as the ageing process continues. They are found in the dermis of the skin and the alveoli of the lungs, both of which are continuously expanding and contracting.

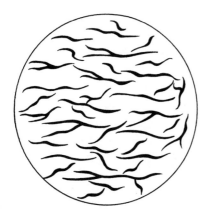

Elastin fibres

Cells within loose connective tissue

The cells found in loose connective tissue may be either *fixed* or *wandering* cells.

Fixed Cells

There are four different kinds of fixed cells. They are:

a) fibroblasts
b) fat cells
c) macrophages
d) mesenchymal cells.

a) Fibroblasts

These are often spindle-shaped with an oval nucleus. Occasionally they may overlap one another like a tiled roof. Fibroblasts produce collagen (from which collagen fibres are formed) and are found close to collagen bundles. Where scar tissue is to be produced, fibroblasts produce extra collagen. This may be at a scar on the skin or internally where muscle has been damaged. The process is known as *fibrosis*.

b) Fat Cells

There are two types of fat cells: white fat cells and brown fat cells. Most of the adipose (fat) cells in

humans are white fat cells. They are formed from a single globule of fat with the nucleus pushed to one end. They are encased in a fine membrane.

i) *White Fat Cells*: These cells are found all over the body, particularly under the skin, around the heart and the kidneys. Females have additional subcutaneous fat deposits in the breasts and buttocks.

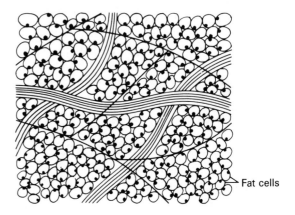

Fat cells

Adipose tissue

ii) *Brown Fat Cells*: These cells get their reddish colour from their abundant blood supply, which also produces a higher metabolic rate. They are found almost exclusively in infants who need to keep a stable body temperature. The body loses them in early childhood.

c) Macrophages

These cells contain a large number of *lysosomes*. They scavenge for all the debris and play an important role in the body's defence against bacterial invasion.

d) Mesenchymal Cells

These are found mostly in embryonic connective tissue. They are thought to produce fibroblasts and fat cells.

Wandering Cells

These include the following:

a) mast cells
b) eosinophil leucocytes
c) lymphocytes and plasma cells
d) monocytes and macrophages
e) blood.

a) Mast Cells

Mast cells contain an anticoagulant substance called *heparin*. They also release *histamine* which dilates small blood vessels and makes their walls more permeable. These cells are therefore important in the body's response to tissue injury.

b) Eosinophil Leucocytes

These cells are produced in bone marrow. They travel around the body in the blood stream. In the healthy human their numbers in connective tissue are small. Their role is to destroy foreign protein. Their numbers rise in cases of hayfever or other allergic conditions.

c) Lymphocytes and Plasma Cells

Lymphocyte cells are the smallest of the wandering cells. Normally their numbers are low in connective tissue. The numbers can dramatically increase and they get larger in size when there is any foreign matter or inflammation. Plasma cells are formed from these cells. The purpose of both types of cells is to destroy foreign protein matter.

d) Monocytes and Macrophages

These are also part of the body's phagocytic system used to destroy foreign matter. They may be found in the alveoli of the lungs where they render harmless any dust particles that are inhaled. They are found particularly in the blood system of the liver and spleen, and in the lymph nodes in the lymphatic system.

e) Blood

This is another form of connective tissue (see Chapter 7).

Dense Connective Tissue

Dense connective tissue is formed mainly from extracellular fibres. It is much firmer than other forms of connective tissue. It does not have its own blood supply. It is nourished by fluid from surrounding tissue. There are four main types:

    hyaline cartilage
    fibrocartilage
    elastic cartilage
    bone.

Hyaline Cartilage

This has a smooth, bluish appearance. It is found at the ends of bones where there are joints. It also forms the costal cartilage (which attaches the ribs to the sternum) and part of the trachea and larynx.

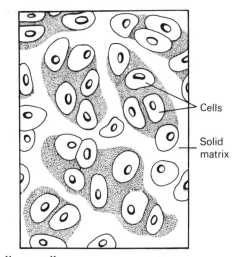

Hyaline cartilage

Fibrocartilage

This consists of a dense mass of white fibres with a solid matrix. It is strong but slightly flexible. It is found in the intervertebral discs which cushion the vertebrae, at the knee in the semilunar cartilage, and at the rims surrounding the hip and shoulder joints.

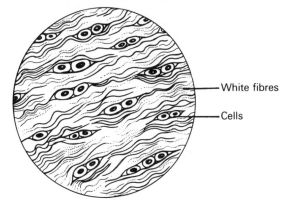

Fibrocartilage

Elastic Cartilage

This consists of yellow elastic fibres in a solid matrix. The soft lobes of the ear and the epiglottis at the back of the mouth are formed from this.

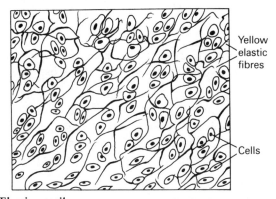

Elastic cartilage

Bone

Bone is the hardest of all forms of connective tissue. It is compsed of:

    25 per cent water
    30 per cent organic matter
    45 per cent inorganic salts.

Bone acts as the body's reservoir for calcium. This is required by muscles for contraction, by nerves for basic functioning, by blood for coagulation and for the formation of bone itself. Bone is constantly being reformed, especially in children, so calcium is an essential mineral in the daily diet. It acts with vitamin D.

Bone is continually being reabsorbed by the phagocytic action of *osteoclasts*. Bone is formed through the action of *osteoblasts* which secrete the collagen found in the matrix. When they are surrounded by the calcified matrix they are called *osteocytes*.

There are two types of bone tissue:

a) compact bone tissue
b) cancellous bone tissue.

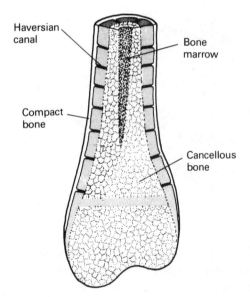

Bone structure

The outer surface of bone is protected by a fine fibrous membrane called *periosteum*. (See Chapter 4.)

a) Compact Bone

This resembles ivory. It is very strong and in the adult, cannot bend. It forms the outer surface of flat bones and the walls of the shaft of long bones.

Compact bone is not a solid mass but is formed from a number of structures called *Haversian systems*. These are cylinders of bone which have a circular canal (*Haversian canal*) running through them. The canals run parallel to the surface of the bone, and carry blood capillaries and lymph vessels. Capillaries bring nourishment to the bone and take away waste material. They also carry minute nerves.

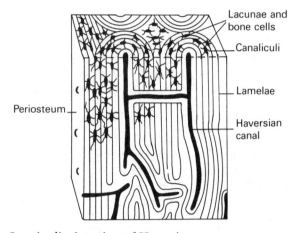

Longitudinal section of Haversian system

Surrounding the Haversian canal are a number of concentric circles called *lamellae* containing bone cells. Between the lamellae are spaces called *lacunae*. These communicate with the Haversian canals and with each other through minute canals called *canaliculi*. They carry lymph to nourish the bone cells. There are small triangular spaces between the Haversian systems called *interstitial lamellae*.

b) Cancellous Bone

Cancellous bone is formed from the same tissue as compact bone. It looks rather like an irregular honeycomb. It is strengthened by a criss-cross of struts and beams.

The purpose of cancellous bone is to make the skeletal frame lighter. It is always covered with a layer of rigid compact bone. The Haversian canals are much larger but there are fewer lamellae.

Bone Marrow

This is a soft, pulpy tissue, found in the interspaces of cancellous bone. It forms the red and white blood cells (see Chapter 4). It is found throughout the bones of the body for the first five years. With age, the red marrow recedes to the ends of the long bones and certain flat bones such as the sternum. This is replaced by a yellow, fatty marrow.

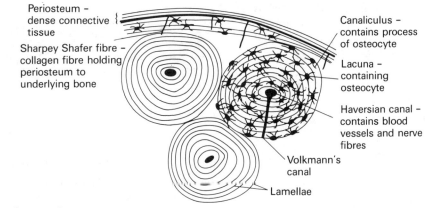

Periosteum – dense connective tissue

Sharpey Shafer fibre – collagen fibre holding periosteum to underlying bone

Canaliculus – contains process of osteocyte

Lacuna – containing osteocyte

Haversian canal – contains blood vessels and nerve fibres

Volkmann's canal

Lamellae

Cross-section of Haversian system

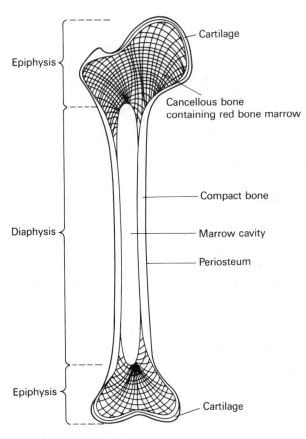

Epiphysis

Diaphysis

Epiphysis

Cartilage

Cancellous bone containing red bone marrow

Compact bone

Marrow cavity

Periosteum

Cartilage

Long bone structure

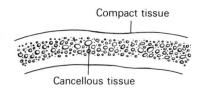

Compact tissue

Cancellous tissue

Flat bone structure

Fascial Tissue

This form of tissue may sometimes be referred to as a *membrane*. There are three types:

mucous membrane
serous membrane
synovial membrane.

Mucous Membrane

This is found lining the nose and mouth, and in the respiratory, alimentary and urino-genital tracts. The membranes are formed from various kinds of epithelial tissue.

The purpose of mucous membranes is to secrete mucus in order to moisten surfaces (such as the lining of the nose) and to provide an absorbing surface (as in the alimentary tract).

Serous Membrane

There are two different kinds of serous membrane:

a) Parietal Serous Membrane

This membrane is formed from squamous epithelial cells. It forms the lining of cavities such as the thorax.

b) Visceral Serous Membrane

This is a fine layer of epithelial cells. It forms a covering around the body's organs such as the pericardium that surrounds the heart.

The main purpose of serous membrane is to stop the organs rubbing against each other and causing friction. The cells secrete a thin serous fluid which helps the organs to move freely against each other.

Synovial Membrane

The ends of bones forming moveable joints are covered with a layer of cartilage. The joint itself is encapsulated by a sheath of fibrous tissue, forming a ligament which holds the joint together: this is known as the *synovial capsule*. The inner lining of this – the *synovial membrane* – secretes a thick fluid for lubricating the joint, called *synovial fluid*.

Muscle Tissue

There are three main types of muscle tissue:

voluntary (striated) muscle
involuntary (smooth) muscle
cardiac muscle.

Voluntary (Striated) Muscle Tissue

These muscles are called *voluntary* because they can be controlled at will. They are under the control of the motor nervous system. They are also known as *skeletal muscles* because they are the ones that cause the bones of the body to move.

Each muscle consists of numerous muscle fibres. The fibres vary in size and length depending on the size of the muscle, but most run the length of the muscle.

Each fibre is formed of a type of cytoplasm called *sarcoplasm*. It contains many flattened nuclei, numerous *mitochondria* and long fine threads called *myofibrils*.

Myofibrils are the contractile part of the muscle fibre. They are composed of still smaller threads called *myofilaments*. These vary in width and shade, giving their overlapping arrangement a pattern of light and dark bands. This is why they are known as *striated* muscles.

The dark myofilaments in a fibre are called 'A' bands. In between the 'A' bands are light bands: these are called 'I' bands. Halfway along each 'I' band is a narrow zone called the 'Z' line. The length between two 'Z' lines is called the *sarcomere*. Within each sarcomere are lengths of thicker myofilaments. These are known as the 'H' zone. This is the part of the fibre that is contracted.

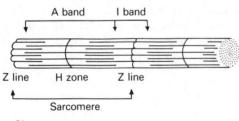

A myofilament

Many myofibrils lie together to form a single muscle fibre. Each fibre is surrounded by a fine membrane called a *sarcolemma*. Between each sarcolemma is a 'T'-shaped tubule containing *interstitial fluid*.

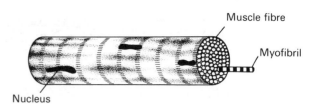

A muscle fibre

Bundles of muscle fibres lying in parallel fashion are called *fasciculi*. Between the fasciculi lies connective tissue called *endomysium*. Each fasciculus is in turn surrounded by a sheath: the *perimysium*. The perimysium is continuous with the tough outer muscle sheath called the *epimysium*. This is extended at the ends of the muscle to form the *tendons*.

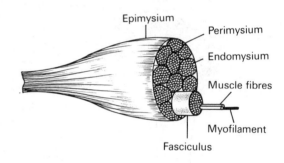

A muscle

Each of the thicker, darker myofilaments ('A' bands) is composed of the proteins *myosin* and *actin*. The thinner, lighter myofilaments ('I' bands) are composed of actin only. Actin contains the two proteins *troponin* and *tropomysin*. When a nerve impulse is sent to the muscle, calcium ions are released into the sarcoplasm. These act with the troponin to shorten the myofilaments in the 'H' zone, thus shortening the sarcomere. When this contraction takes place over the whole muscle, the muscle gets shorter and fatter at the *belly* or centre.

Energy is supplied to the muscle fibres by the blood in the form of *adenosine triphosphate* (ATP), creating phosphate and glycogen. In order to create energy for movement, oxygen is also taken from the blood supply. It oxidises the glucose. If further energy is required, as when strenuous bouts of exercise are performed, *anaerobic glycolysis* is produced. This does not require oxygen to produce energy, but it does produce an oxygen debt. *Lactic acid* in the body then stimulates increased respiration so that the oxygen debt is repaid.

Involuntary (Smooth) Muscle Tissue

Involuntary muscles cannot be controlled at will. They are controlled by the autonomic nervous system. They are found in organs such as the walls of the blood vessels, the respiratory and alimentary tracts and the urino-genital organs. They may sometimes be referred to as *visceral muscles*.

The fibres are spindle-shaped and have only one nucleus. They have no distinct sarcolemma. The bundles of fibres are usually found lying in layers so as to form a wall for the organ concerned

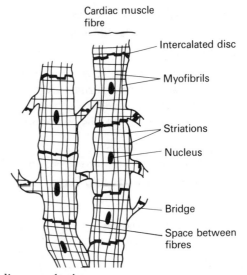

Cardiac muscle tissue

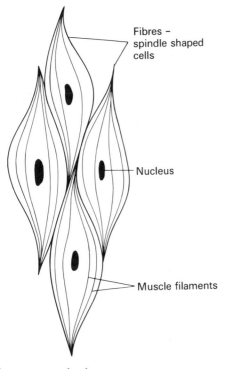

Involuntary muscle tissue

Cardiac Muscle Tissue

These muscle fibres are only found in the walls of the heart. They resemble the involuntary muscle in structure but have the striation of the voluntary muscles. However, cardiac muscle has a special property not found in either of the other two types of muscle. It has the ability to contract rhythmically, independently of its nerve supply.

The fibres are cylindrical with a branch connecting them to another fibre at an *intercalated disc*. The group of fibres between each disc have a single central nucleus. The intercalated disc allows the contraction of one fibre to stimulate the contraction of the adjacent fibre.

Nervous Tissue

Movement or function of any organ is governed by the nervous system. There are two kinds of nerve cell:

>   neurons
>   non-excitable tissue cells.

Neurons

The nerve cells are called *neurons*. They vary in size from being some of the smallest cells in the body to the largest.

Each neuron contains a cytoplasm called *perikaryon*. The bulbous part of the cell body is called a *soma*. It has a central nucleus. There are several golgi bodies and lysosomes whose function is to remove waste material. Once it is formed, the neuron is usually incapable of cell division.

A number of processes are given off from the soma. There is one long process called the *axon*. The cytoplasm within the axon is called *axoplasm*. It is covered by a membrane called the *axolemma*. Some axon are covered by a sheath of fatty material which gives them a white appearance. This is called a *myelin sheath* and gives these cells the name *white matter* (*myelinated fibres*). The function of the myelin sheath is to act as an insulator and to speed the flow of nerve impulses along the nerve pathway.

Some neurons do not have a myelin sheath. They are known as *non-myelinated* nerve fibres or *grey matter*. They are most often to be found in the autonomic nervous system, part of the central nervous system and in the fine sensory peripheral nerves (see Chapter 6).

At intervals along the axon, there are breaks in the myelin sheath. These help the impulses to travel faster along the nerve.

The shaft of the axon is covered by a fine membrane called the *neurilemma*. This is formed from *Schwann* cells. It works as an inverted tubing to give protection and to assist in the transmission of impulses.

The end of the axon divides into several branches. The ends of these are called *presynaptic knobs* or *end feet*.

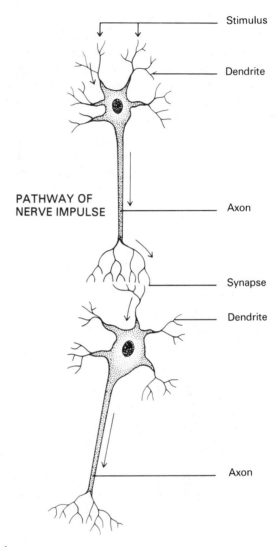

PATHWAY OF NERVE IMPULSE

A synapse

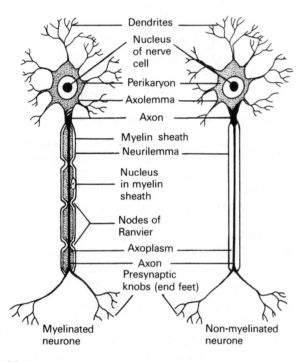

Neurons

Also given off from the soma are a number of small dividing processes called *dendrites*.

Nerve impulses are carried along the dendrite towards the nerve cell itself. They are then carried forward to the next cell along the axon.

Where the dendrite of one neuron and the axon of the next meet, there is a minute space called a *synapse*. Impulses are transmitted along a nerve by a chemical action. When a nerve impulse is received at an axon it triggers the release of chemical transmitters such as *acetylcholine*. Other chemical transmitters are believed to include *noradrenalin*, *dopamine* and *5 hydroxy-tryptamine*. These stimulate the dendrites of the next neuron to accept the impulse. The chemical is then neutralised and the axon relaxes.

Non-Excitable Tissue Cells
A different form of connective tissue supports the nerve cells of the brain and spinal cord. It is called *neuroglia*. There are three main types: oligodendro-cytes, astrocytes, and microglia.

These neuroglia, together with the Schwann cells are classified as non-excitable cells because they do not transmit impulses.

Special Characteristics
Nervous tissue has two special characteristics. They are: *irritability* and *conductivity*.

Irritability
Nerves are able to respond to stimuli from:

1 Outside the body, e.g. touch, sight, etc.
2 Inside the body, e.g. an increase in carbon dioxide in the blood may increase voluntary movement.

Conductivity

Nerves are able to transmit an impulse from:

1 One part of the brain to another, or to the spinal cord.
2 The brain to voluntary muscles to cause a contraction and so move a joint.
3 The brain to involuntary muscles to stimulate secretion of glands.
4 Muscles and joints so as to coordinate balance.
5 Organs of the body so as to maintain body functions.
6 Outside the body through the special senses of sight, sound, taste, smell and touch.
7 Outside the body through the sensory nerve endings stimulated by heat and cold, rough and smooth, etc.

METABOLISM

This is a chemical process that takes place in the cells. There are two types:

1 *Anabolism*: this is the build-up of complex compounds from simple ones; resulting in growth and storage of energy. (Energy may also be stored in the form of ATP: see page 14).
2 *Catabolism*: this is the breakdown of complex compounds into simple ones; releasing energy. For example, when 'food' is oxidised in the cells, energy is released in the form of heat.

The body needs to replace millions of cells every minute. This takes place through cell division, which requires energy. Energy is also required to maintain body temperature at approximately 37 °C or 98.4 °F.

Energy may be expressed in units of heat as a *calorie*, or in units of work as a *joule*. A calorie may be described as the amount of heat required to raise the temperature of 1 gram of water through 1 degree Celsius.

1 calorie = 4186 joules (J)

Joules are sometimes counted as kilojoules (kJ) so that 1 calorie might be said to equal 4.186 kJ.

Food, in the form of carbohydrates, proteins or fats, may be expressed as calories or kilojoules per gram.

The minimum amount of energy required by the body is called the *basal metabolic rate* (BMR). It is higher in men than in women of the same height, weight and age. Men will therefore require more energy-producing foods to achieve the same outcome.

Metabolism of Carbohydrates

When carbohydrates are digested they are changed into *monosaccharides*, mainly in the form of glucose. This is absorbed into the blood system from the small intestine. Some of this glucose will remain in the blood and travel around the body to provide the energy needed by the various cells for their replacement. Glucose provides energy for all the activities that take place in the liver, as well as being stored there as *glycogen*. Any excess glucose is converted into fat and deposited around the body.

Metabolism of Protein

Unlike carbohydrate, protein is not stored in the body. Protein is changed into twenty *amino acids* which are used for synthesis by the cells. Any excess amino acids are converted by the liver into *urea* and expelled by the body.

Metabolism of Fat

Fats and oils are absorbed from the intestines and carried eventually to the liver. Here they may be stored as glycogen. The liver also changes them into cholesterol. This is carried in the bloodstream and is used particularly to synthesise cell membranes.

THE IMMUNE SYSTEM

The immune system is the body's defence against viral or bacterial invaders. It is aided by several forms of natural protection that serve to prevent bacteria entering the body in the first instance.

Natural Protection

The human baby is born with a form of innate immunity, sometimes called 'natural immunity'. This does not protect the individual against any specific infection, and is not thought to last for very long.

There are, however, three other forms of protection against invading bacteria:
   mechanical
   chemical
   thermal.

Mechanical Protection

The skin is a very effective barrier. When it is unbroken, it effectively stops micro-organisms from entering the body (see Chapter 3). The mucous membranes of the respiratory and alimentary tracts form a different kind of protection. When dust enters the respiratory tract, the cilia hairs waft it back to the nasal cavity. The peristaltic action of the alimentary tract moves food along its length. Because of this movement, bacteria are dislodged and so cannot increase in number and therefore cause an infection.

Chemical Protection

The skin also acts as a chemical protection. The sebum secreted by the sebaceous glands and the sweat secreted by the sweat glands both have an antebacterial effect. Certain enzymes such as *muramidase* found in tears can break down bacteria, as can the acid found in the stomach. The bacterial enzyme *lysozyme* is present in substances secreted within the respiratory system.

Certain cells in the body act against invading bacteria. They are called *phagocytic* cells. *Leucocytes* and *macrophages* are both types of phagocytic cells. The leucocytes circulate in the blood system. They engulf and then break down bacteria. Macrophages circulate in the blood stream and are also found in connective tissue; they secrete an enzyme called *lysosome*. This attaches its own cell walls to certain bacteria, the enzyme then enters and breaks down the bacteria. The process is called *lysis*.

Some cells, when attacked by a virus, produce a protein called *interferon*. This can prohibit the virus from reproducing itself, by interacting with its RNA. In some instances interferon may change the membrane of the cell under attack so that the virus cannot gain access to it.

Thermal Protection

A number of viruses and bacteria, but not all, are unable to exist for long in a cold environment. They are therefore unable to live outside a human host.

Acquired Immunity

Immunity can be acquired against a specific organism such as measles or tuberculosis. This involves the action of antibodies.

Antibodies

Human cells are capable of recognising other cells from their own body. They can also recognise cells that are not of their own body. These foreign cells are often recognised by their different carbohydrates or glycoproteins on their outside walls, known as *antigens*. The antigens cause the body to produce *antibodies*. Each antibody will only recognise one specific form of antigen.

Antigens stimulate the immune system into producing antibodies for fighting off the specific disease. This will be through the action of B-lymphocytes or T-lymphocytes. B-lymphocytes are formed in the bone marrow, and then stored in the lymph nodes or spleen. T-lymphocytes depend on the thymus gland for their development. If a young person has an underdeveloped thymus, they will have few T-lymphocytes and therefore a lower resistance to infection.

In some instances the B- or T-lymphocytes fail to recognise the body's own cells. They will attack them as well as cells having a similar antigen and so leave the body open to a wide variety of infections. This condition is known as an auto-immune deficiency syndrome (AIDS).

When cells produce antibodies which combine with antigens, the process is called *humoral* immune response. Occasionally harmless antigens such as pollen may produce both antibodies and antigen-antibody complexes. In the case of pollen, this can cause a severe reaction such as asthma or hayfever.

There are two ways of obtaining acquired immunity:
  actively
  passively.

Actively Acquired Immunity

This occurs when the body manufactures its own antibodies. The immunity may be acquired by three methods:
  clinical disease
  subclinical disease
  vaccination.

Clinical Disease

Immunity can be acquired by actually having a specific disease, such as measles. The body will produce antibodies to overcome the disease. Some of these antibodies will remain in the body. If the body is attacked again by the same specific disease, the antibodies will overcome it so that that person will not have the disease a second time.

Subclinical Disease

In some instances a subclinical infection may take

place. A person may be exposed to a specific disease but not show any reaction to it. The body's immune system however, will produce antibodies to overcome it and so sensitise the body for future protection.

Vaccination

Immunity can be acquired by having a vaccination. Specific viruses or bacteria are cultivated in a laboratory and then 'killed' by means of heat or chemicals. These are then injected into the body which then manufactures its own antibodies to the disease.

Passively Acquired Immunity

In this case, antibodies are passed into the body from another source, e.g. when human or animal serum already containing antibodies is injected into a person. The serum is taken from people who are recovering from the specific disease and therefore have the antibodies in their blood. The serum may be given *prophylactically*, i.e. to prevent a person catching a specific disease such as influenza. It may also be given *therapeutically*, i.e. to treat a person who already has the disease.

Chapter 3

The Skin

The skin is the largest organ in the body. It weighs approximately 7 pounds (3 kilos) and covers the whole of the body. It is thickest on the palms of the hands and soles of the feet. It is thinnest on the eyelids. There are two main types of skin:

    glabrous skin
    hairy skin.

Glabrous Skin

This is found only on the palms of the hands and soles of the feet. The surface has a number of ridges and grooves. This type of skin has a thicker epidermis, a greater number of tactile nerve endings and shows an absence of hair follicles and sebaceous glands.

Hairy Skin

This is found on the rest of the body. It has fewer tactile nerve endings but produces both hair follicles and sebaceous glands.

LAYERS OF THE SKIN

The skin consists of three layers:
    the epidermis
    the dermis
    the subcutis.

The Epidermis

This is the most superficial layer. It is formed from two distinct cellular processes. These both contain several different types of cell each forming a layer which evolves from the layer below. They are: the *keratinisation (horny) zone* and the *germinative zone*.

Cells generated in the germinative zone are pushed upwards through the three layers of the epidermis, losing their nuclei and dying as they near the surface of the skin.

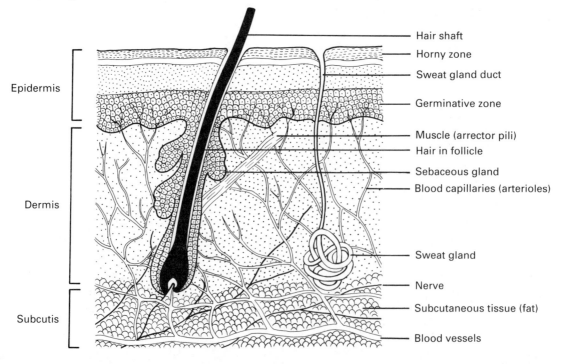

Layers of the skin

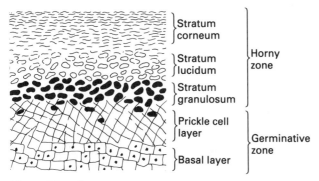

Stratum corneum
Stratum lucidum
Stratum granulosum
} Horny zone

Prickle cell layer
Basal layer
} Germinative zone

The epidermis

For additional details of the different types of cell, see Chapter 1.

The Keratinisation (Horny) Zone
This is divided into three layers:
    the stratum corneum
    the stratum lucidum
    the stratum granulosum.

The Stratum Corneum (cornified layer)
This is the surface layer of the skin. It consists of thin, flat, dead *squamous* cells whose *protoplasm* has been changed into a horny substance called *keratin*. They have completely lost their nuclei. They lie flattened and overlapping one another. They adhere closely together to prevent tissue fluid loss from the body and to keep out harmful bacteria and fluids, making the skin a virtually watertight membrane. The cells become more loosely packed as they move nearer the surface of the skin. They are eventually shed as dry, flaky dead cells. The life span of epidermal cells is approximately 28 to 30 days. About half of this time is spent in the stratum corneum. They lie on top of:

The Stratum Lucidum
This is found mostly in the areas of glabrous skin. The granular layer from below has become thickened and hardened. It is composed of many closely packed cells of a distinctive shape. Traces of flattened nuclei may still be visible. As they are clear, some light may pass through these cells. This layer links the living cells of the granular layer to the non-nucleated cells of the horny layer above. It lies above:

The Stratum Granulosum (granular layer)
This consists of living cells of a definite shape. They each contain a nucleus surrounded by numerous granules of a substance called *keratohyalin*. As these cells move upwards through the epidermis, they are converted into *keratin* by an enzyme. During *keratinisation*, moisture is lost from the cells as they lose their nuclei. They then become the horny outer layer (stratum corneum). In the areas of hairy skin, this layer is often transformed directly into the stratum corneum.

Below the keratinisation zone lies the germinative zone.

The Germinative Zone
This consists of two layers: the *stratum spinosum* and the *basal layer*.

The Stratum Spinosum
This is sometimes called the *prickle cell layer* because of the prickly appearance of the cells called *keratinocytes*. They are polygonal in shape and contain a nucleus. They are connected to the adjoining cells by thin fibres. As they are pushed upwards by the new cells that are forming beneath them, they become flattened and form a new layer. The layer below is called:

The Basal Layer
This may sometimes be called the *malpighian layer*. It consists of a single layer of cells firmly attached to the underlying dermis.

The basal cells contain a nucleus. They are constantly dividing by mitosis to produce new cells. When skin is superficially cut or damaged, it is 'repaired' in this layer. The new cells, which have fine filaments, constantly push the older cells upwards. From the time of their formation until they are discarded, these cells last about six weeks.

Between these cells lie specialised cells called *melanocytes* (*melanoblasts*). They secrete a brown pigment called *melanin*, a protein-like part of the amino-acid *tyrosine*. Its production is controlled partly by genetic inheritance and partly by hormonal secretions. The stimulation of melanocytes can be increased by exposure to ultraviolet rays. This can have a self-protecting effect by thickening the skin. Melanin increases the brown colour of the skin. Black or brown skin produces far more melanin than white skin from the same number of melanocytes. An absence of melanin produces totally white hair and pink eyes with poor vision, a condition known as *albinism*.

The Dermis (Corium)
This is sometimes called the *true skin*. It lies below the epidermis and is constantly being renewed. It is thicker in some areas such as the palms of the hands and soles of the feet and is very fine on the eyelids. The dermis contains blood capillaries, lymph canals, nerves and nerve endings, sweat glands, hair follicles, small muscles and sebaceous glands. The bulk of the dermal tissue is formed from collagen tissue. Two

other proteins, elastin and reticulin, are also found. They give the skin its flexibility and strength. They are synthesised by fibroblasts which are the most numerous cells found in the dermis.

The dermis consists of two main layers: *the papillary layer* and *the reticular layer*.

The Papillary Layer

This is the superficial dermal layer. It consists of numerous conical projections called *papillae*. Each papilla consists of fine fibril tissue and a few elastic fibres. Some may contain tactile nerve endings. On the palms of the hands and the soles of the feet, the papillae are arranged in parallel lines in elevated patterns to show the characteristic finger prints (they are less numerous in other parts of the body). The ducts of sweat glands pass outwards between these ridges. The ridges and furrows fall into an irregular pattern in folds at the joints to allow for movement. They protect against continuous friction, help to prevent slippage when holding an object and allow one to walk without continually slipping.

The Reticular Layer

This consists mainly of interfacing bands of strong, white, fibrous reticular tissue and some yellow elastic fibres. The yellow fibres atrophy and lose much of their elasticity with age or from excessive ultraviolet light, making the skin lined and wrinkled. For the most part, all the bundles of fibres lie in parallel bands. The direction that the bundles of fibres take are known as the *cleavage lines*. This is important in surgery. If an incision is made along these lines it should heal leaving only a very fine scar. If the incision is made across the cleavage lines, the scar is likely to be broader. Generally the lines are horizontal on the trunk, neck and limbs and vertical on the shoulders and buttocks.

If the skin is stretched, as in pregnancy or obesity, the fibrous bands may become stretched and rupture, forming scar tissue which looks like white or silver streaks. They are commonly called *stretch marks*.

The Subcutis (Hypodermis)

This is the deepest layer of the skin. It is formed from loose connective tissue separating the skin from the underlying muscle tissue. This permits the skin to move easily over the underlying tissues. An ample supply of blood and lymph vessels, nerve endings and fat cells are found here. The fat cells act as a storage depot and are more numerous in women, giving them a more feminine, rounded appearance. The fat also helps reduce heat loss.

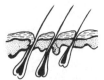

65 hairs

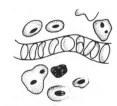

9,500,000 cells

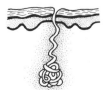

95–100 sebaceous glands

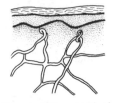

19 yards (17 metres) of blood vessels

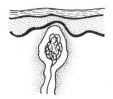

650 sweat glands

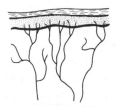

78 yards (70 metres) of nerves

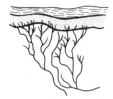

78 sensory apparatuses for heat

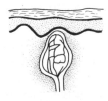

19,500 sensory cells at the ends of nerve fibres

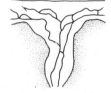

1,300 nerve endings to record pain

160–165 pressure pads for the perception of tactile stimuli

13 sensory apparatuses for cold

Structures in the skin (approximate numbers in one square inch)

COMPONENTS OF THE SKIN

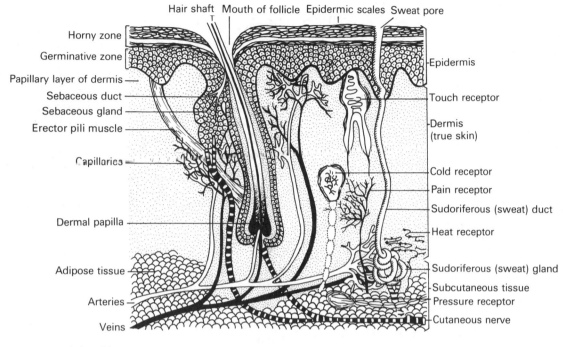

Components of the skin

The dermis contains:

Capillary Blood Vessels

A fine network of capillary blood vessels (arterioles) supplies oxygen and nutrients to the skin. Deoxygenated blood is carried away by a fine meshwork of venules to the larger venous system and thence back to the lungs. These blood vessels also play an important part in regulating the temperature of the body. When the body temperature is high, blood flows near the surface of the skin where it loses heat. When the body temperature is low, the arterioles constrict so that the blood flow to the cooler skin is restricted. When the skin surface is cut, certain components in the blood form a clot. This prevents further escape of blood and prevents bacteria entering the system.

Lymphatic Vessels

Lymph vessels (or canals) drain away waste particles that are often too large for the veins to carry. They begin as lymph spaces in the papillary layer and then form lymph vessels which eventually link up with those from all parts of the body. Lymph glands are one of the body's main defences against the spread of infection.

Nerves

Much of the body's sensory 'information' originates from the sensory nerves found in the skin. Nerve impulses are transmitted through a fine network of both myelinated (white) and non-myelinated (grey) nerve fibres. The nerves are not evenly distributed. For example, there are far more in areas such as the fingertips than on the upper arms. The tactile nerve endings respond to the stimulus of touch, pain, temperature, etc. They may also respond directly to some chemicals such as those in certain washing powders. Sympathetic nerves supply other skin components such as the blood vessels, arrector pili muscles and sweat glands.

Sweat (Sudorific) Glands

These glands are found all over the body. There are two kinds: the *eccrine glands* and the *aprocrine glands*.

Eccrine Glands

These are present in all parts of the dermis. They are most numerous in the palms of the hands and the soles of the feet, with fewer on the neck and back. They vary in size, being largest in areas where sweating is greatest, such as the axilla (arm-pit) and groin. The main part (or body) of the gland lies like a coiled tube. It has a duct which opens onto the surface of the skin known as the sweat pore. The glands may be activated into producing sweat by emotional tension, heat, pain, etc. They are supplied by sympathetic nerve fibres and also by the capillary blood system. One of their main functions is to control body temperatures. They secrete a thin watery fluid which evaporates on the surface of the skin, helping to keep it cool. Another function is to expel waste materials such as salt and urea.

Water secreted from the epidermal spaces is continually evaporated from the skin surface without making the skin wet; this is known as 'insensible perspiration'. It becomes part of the *acid mantle*, which is a film formed from several body fluids. It assists the skin to remain at the correct acidity.

Apocrine Glands

These glands are larger than eccrine glands and produce a thicker secretion. They only begin to function at puberty. Their ducts open into hair follicles. They are mainly found at the axilla, the genital and anal areas, and the nipples. They may be activated by emotional tension, pain or sexual activity. The sweat produced by these glands is an odourless milky secretion. When it starts to decompose through bacterial action a characteristically unpleasant odour will prevail. They do not respond as much as eccrine glands to a change in body temperature but are controlled by the activity of the sympathetic nervous system.

Sebaceous Glands

These are found all over the skin except for the palms of the hands and the soles of the feet. They are found in great numbers on the scalp, face and sometimes the back. The glands are formed of epidermal cells and usually, but not always, open into a hair follicle. They can also extend directly to the skin surface, especially around the nose and mouth. They secrete an oily substance called sebum which helps to keep the skin supple and the hair soft. Sebum also has a bacterial effect through acting as part of the acid mantle. The glands are stimulated by hormonal action, especially androgens (which stimulate the growth of male secondary sex characteristics). Therefore there is little activity in these glands until puberty.

Too little sebum results in dry, brittle hair, and dry, flaky skin. Too much gives the skin and hair a greasy appearance. If the pores become blocked with sebum or sweat, blackheads, whiteheads and other conditions can arise.

Hair

Hair can be found over nearly all the body except the palms of the hands and soles of the feet. It varies in length, colour and texture in different areas of the same body and in different ethnic groups.

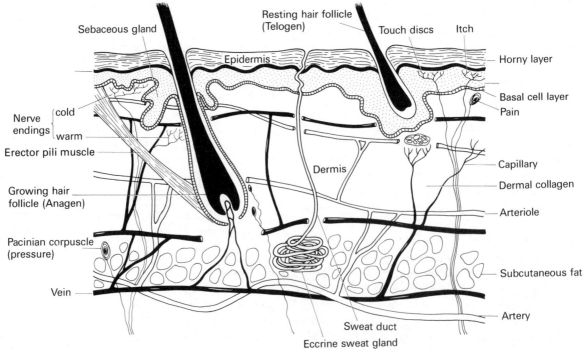

Hair

Each hair lies in a depression of epidermal cells called a *hair follicle*. The follicle is supplied by blood vessels and nerve endings. Hair is formed here in a layer of germinal cells (see Chapter 9). The part of the hair lying above the skin is the *shaft*, while that lying within the follicle is the *root*. The lower end of the root expands to become the hair *bulb*. Below this is a projection of dermal cells: the papillae.

Nails

These are plates of horny cells found on the dorsal surfaces of the fingers and toes. The part of the nail extending beyond the digit is called the *free edge*. The main part of the nail is the *body*, which is firmly attached to the underlying nail bed. The root is embedded in a groove of skin. Below this is the growing area or *matrix*. A fold of skin at each side of the nail (*nail wall*) extends along the base to form the cuticle (see Chapter 9).

SKIN COLOUR

This can be determined by the presence of different pigments or other factors found in the skin. The distribution varies throughout the body and with age, genetic and racial differences.

1 *Melanin*, a brown pigment, is produced mainly by the melanocytes in the basal layer of the epidermis.
2 *Melanoid* is a similar substance to melanin, and is found throughout the epidermis.
3 *Carotene* is a yellow/orange pigment produced in the horny layer and in adipose (fat) cells of the dermis.
4 *Haemoglobin*, contained in the vascular system, is a purple colour.
5 *Oxyhaemoglobin*, a red colour, is also contained in the vascular system.

An absence of pigmentation results in albinism, whereby patches of skin or the total skin area remain white.

PHYSICAL DIFFERENCES DUE TO ETHNIC INFLUENCE

Apart from the obvious differences of skin and hair colour within ethnic groups, relatively little is known about the skin structure or the body functions which influence it. Skin colours range from white to yellow, light to dark, brown to black with varying overtones of bronze, copper, or grey. The variations depend on the amount of melanin produced together with the other colourant agents. Colour can be due to race, geographical origin and genetic structure. Local as well as global similarities and differences can occur.

It is said that dark skins absorb more heat energy than white skins. Light skins have a slightly higher body temperature than dark under desert conditions. The extremities (fingers, toes) of people with black skin cool much more rapidly than those with light skin. An eskimo's skin takes longer to cool than the average light skin.

Dark skin synthesises less vitamin D than white skin in temperate climes. Light skin generally shows the ageing process earlier than dark skin.

The epidermis of black skin may frequently tend to shed grey shiny scales, though generally the skin is velvety to the touch. The dermis of black skin is often slightly thicker than that of light skin.

In black skin the sudorific (sweat) glands are larger and more numerous. Their number is increased still further in the Indian races, hence their ability to withstand heat better than the light-skinned people of Europe or the Far East. The secretion from the eccrine glands is likely to have a pH of 3.5 to 5.6 (see page 26). Lactic acids, fatty acids and some ammonia are secreted, helping to maintain the softness of the skin. The secretion from the apocrine glands is more likely to be neutral or even alkaline. This can neutralise the acid mantle so enabling bacteria to enter the skin. Sebaceous glands are larger and more numerous in dark skin. As well as opening into the hair follicle they open directly onto the surface of the skin. The secretion is likely to contain more fatty material than that of light skin. However, the skin is not oily (as light skin would be) because it is thought to be mixed with a residue of cutaneous fluid. Extra care should therefore be taken when cleansing dark skin, especially around the hairline.

Whereas light skin will blanch where there is a cut, scarring or skin eruption, black skin will take on a darker, purplish hue.

The nails of dark-skinned people may have coloured linear streaks.

Hair type varies with race, culture, environment and genetic structures. The natural colour can be anywhere from white (blonde) to black with many variations. It can be straight, wavy, helical or spiral. In cross-sections it may be round or ovoid. There is generally less hair distributed on the body of people with black skin, than on those with light skin.

FUNCTIONS OF THE SKIN

Protection
The skin acts as a protective covering for internal structures. The fat cells of the subcutis protect the body against blows and falls. The horny layer acts as a barrier against bacteria and micro-organisms. It also prevents water from entering the body and body fluids, electrolytes, etc. from leaving the body. The basal layer protects the body from the harmful effects of ultraviolet rays. Sebum, as part of the acid mantle, acts as a slightly bactericidal agent. The darker the melanic pigmentation, the greater the protection from the sun's radiation.

Sensation
The skin contains many tactile nerve endings. The brain is made aware of the different stimuli of pain, cold, heat, etc. experienced in any part of the body through the sensory nervous system; giving an awareness of surroundings. The nerve endings (receptors) are found at different levels in the dermis according to their specific function. Those of touch lie close to the surface. Cold is felt a little deeper while warmth is felt by still deeper receptors. Pain is felt by receptors at varying levels.

Heat Regulation
The skin helps to regulate and control the body temperature at 36.8 °C (98.4 °F) through a number of different ways. Insulation occurs when the body gets cold. The capillaries constrict so that the warmer blood remains deeper in the body. The arrector pili muscles raise the hair, trapping a layer of air against the surface skin; and the sweat glands become less active. As a result of the cold stimulation, the skeletal muscles go into an involuntary shiver.

When the body becomes too hot, fluid from the sebaceous glands and epidermal spaces is secreted onto the surface of the skin. As this fluid evaporates it has a cooling effect. The capillaries dilate (expand), allowing the blood to flow nearer the cooler skin surface and thus lose heat. There is more evaporation from black skin than light skin, which assists it in keeping cool in high temperatures. However, light skin has a higher cold tolerance.

Secretion
Sebum is secreted by the sebaceous glands. It helps to maintain suppleness of the skin and softness of the hair. It also acts as a bactericide and contributes to the acid mantle having a pH of between 5.0 and 5.6.

Sweat is secreted by the eccrine and apocrine glands. This helps in regulating body temperature. It also contributes to the acid mantle.

Elimination
Sweating helps the body dispose of some waste materials such as urea and lactic acid.

Absorption
Thin fluids such as aqueous solutions are not readily absorbed through the skin. Some products such as oil or fatty-based substances may be absorbed in small quantities. Some drugs are administered in this manner.

Storage
The subcutaneous layer acts as one of the main deposits of fat in the body, while skin tissues contain up to 15 per cent of the body's fluid.

Vitamin D
Formation of vitamin D takes place in the skin. Ultraviolet rays act on a substance called ergosterol which together with phosphorus and calcium assists in the formation of bone.

DISORDERS OR ABNORMALITIES OF THE SKIN

Erythema A localised reddening of the skin caused by dilation of the capillaries.

Pigmentation The natural colour of the skin due to the amount of melanin, melanoid, or carotene produced in the skin. Bile, as when jaundiced, and certain drugs can alter the natural skin colour.

Naevus (Nevus) This term denotes an area of skin discolouration due to pigmentation. The most common are:
Araneous (Spider) A bright red spot caused by dilated arterioles. It is surrounded by a fine network of blood vessels which resembles a spider's web.
Haemangioma: Capillary (Port wine stain) An area of raised, dark red skin caused by dilated blood vessels. It is present at birth and is permanent.
Haemangioma: Cavernous (Strawberry mark) Also an area of raised, red skin, this looks rather like a dark red strawberry. It is caused by the enlargement of locally superficial blood vessels. Formed in infancy, it usually resolves itself before puberty.

Vitiligo Patches of milky white skin in areas of normal pigmentation. This is more noticeable in darker skin. It may be caused by a virus or over-exposure to ultraviolet.

Albinism Pale pink (white) skin, white hair, and pink eyes, due to the absence of pigmentation in the skin. It may cover the total body area, or affect some parts only.

Chloasma Patches of brown skin in areas of normal pigmentation caused by an increase of melanin. It is often associated with pregnancy, the 'Pill', advancing age, certain chemicals (e.g. perfume) and sunlight (ultraviolet rays).

Macule A small area of different colour to the surrounding skin.

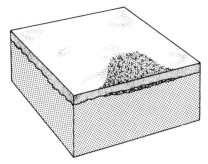

A macule

Papule A small, firm raised lesion.

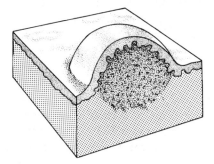

A papule

Nodule A larger raised lesion formed under the skin.

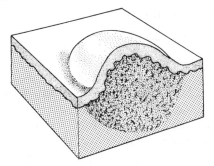

A nodule

Wheal A slightly raised lesion, white at the centre, pale red at the edge.

Blister A pocket containing fluid.

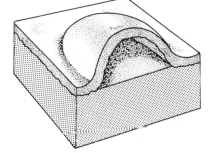

A blister

Vesicle A very small blister.

Bulla A larger blister.

Pustule A blister of any size containing pus.

Scale Loosened horny cells which may be dry or oily.

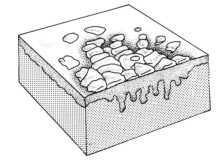

Scale

Crust Dried sebum on the surface of the skin.

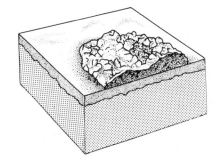

Crust

Erosion A partial loss of epidermal skin.

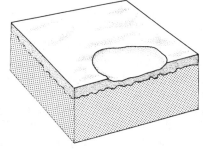

Erosion

Ulcer A total loss of epidermal skin with an inflamed base. The dermal skin may also be eroded.

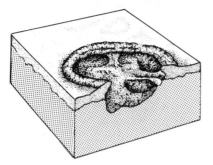

An ulcer

Fissure A crack or split in the epidermis.

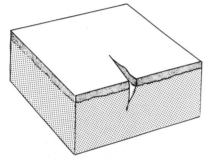

Fissure

Atrophy A wasting away of tissue with depigmentation.

Hypertrophy An increase in tissue growth.

Keloid Scar tissue which is thickened and hard.

Melanocytic Naevus (Mole) An area of elevated skin. They may be soft or hard, smooth or rough, light or dark in colour. Some may produce hair. This is a very common condition. Most moles are benign; if they are irritated they may bleed, spread rapidly and become cancerous.

Wart An elevation of the skin resulting from over-production of prickle cells, caused by a virus (see Chapter 14).

Skin Tags Small, stalk-shaped tags of loose fibrous tissue often found on the neck in middle-aged people.

Wen A benign cyst resulting from the retention of sebum.

Comedones Commonly called blackheads. In some instances they may be formed by sebum trapped in the pores. The sebum dries and hardens. The surface becomes black through oxidisation. Melanocyte cells, which produce the pigment melanin, can also cause this blackening. These are sometimes found in the upper part of the hair follicle. If the follicle becomes clogged with sebum, some of the melanin becomes mixed with it, giving the sebum a dark appearance.

Closed Comedones The comedones are formed and then enclosed by a layer of keratinous skin.

Milia Commonly called whiteheads. They are formed by sebum trapped under the skin. They remain white because the surface is not exposed to the air.

Seborrhoea An excessive secretion of sebum by the sebaceous glands which often become enlarged. The skin becomes very oily and has a shiny appearance. The pores may become blocked causing comedones. These may become inflamed causing pustules to occur. Severe cases may lead to acne.

Acne Vulgaris One of the most common skin conditions. It can be either a chronic or acute condition. It affects the sebaceous glands which become inflamed due to infection. It is often found on the face, neck, back or chest. The condition is most common at puberty. Often the earlier it appears, the longer it lasts. The condition usually disappears by the time the person is 25 years old. A possible cause could be an increase in the sex hormones. The condition may be made worse by such factors as stress, diet, or certain clothing fabrics, e.g. nylon or irritating materials (wool or fur). It starts as seborrhoea with comedones and closed comedones. Some of these develop into pustules which may rupture and so spread infection. The epidermis may thicken with cysts forming. Scars and 'pitting' can occur. The surface of the skin can become thickened, uneven and have a greasy appearance.

Rosacea Acne rosacea is not to be confused with true acne. This is a chronic congestion of the superficial blood vessels. It usually only affects the centre panel of the face and the forehead. It is most commonly found in women of menopausal age. The skin of the area may appear thickened and have open pores and broken veins. Papules and pustules may occasionally be present. This condition may be exaggerated by anything causing vasodilation, e.g. heat, sunshine, spiced foods, alcohol and stress.

Dermatitis An inflammation of the skin caused by external factors. It may start as an erythema with itching or irritation. Papules and vesicles can appear, burst and form a crust. Oedema may also be present. It can effect both sexes, at any age in any climate. There are many causes including: *Plants* (tomato, daffodil, strawberry, ivy, etc.); *Wood* (teak, ebony); *Drugs* (penicillin, antihistamine etc.); *Clothing* (certain dyes, wool, synthetic materials, metal zips etc.); *Cosmetics* (lipsticks, nail polish, some hair dyes etc.); *Chemicals* (detergents, petroleum and its by-products etc.).

Eczema Similar to dematitis, but of unknown origin. There are four different types: *Atopic* (hereditary, relating to asthma, hay fever and urticaria); *Infantile*; *Childhood*; *Adult*.

Herpes Simplex (Cold sore) This often heralds a cold. Blisters form, usually around the mouth. These break and become crusted. This can be accompanied by a sharp, tingling sensation. A cold sore will often re-appear in the same place. It is originally caused by a virus.

Psoriasis This starts as an area of erythema which becomes covered with silvery scales. It can then become ulcerated. The area affected may be just a small patch (as at the elbow) or a greater part of the body, including the nails and scalp. Although it can look unpleasant, it is not contagious. The cause is generally unknown but it is often hereditary.

Boil An acute inflammation of glands or hair follicles where pus occurs. It is caused by a staphylococcal (bacterial) infection.

Carbuncle A deeper-seated infection than a boil, this may have more than one septic focal point.

Abscess An acute bacterial infection, often at the site of a foreign body. There will be a redness and localised swelling. When it is ready to burst, the skin becomes very thin and turns a bluish-red.

Urticaria (Hives or nettle rash) An allergy marked by the eruption of wheals with severe itching. It may disappear, only to reappear elsewhere. It can be caused by certain foods, drugs, insect bites, pollens, etc. In certain instances, stress has been found to cause this condition.

Skin Cancer This can affect those areas of the body that are most often exposed to the sun. It may start as a pale lesion, a red patch or a coloured mole. If there is any rapid change in appearance – an increase in size, a change in colour or the onset of ulceration – it may indicate a skin cancer.
Skin cancer can occur in various forms such as:
Rodent Ulcer This causes destruction to organs by eating into the tissues. The most common sites are the angles of the eyes, the hairline and the sides of the nose. It is caused by a malignant growth of basal cells. In the early stages the tumour is slow-growing. In later stages it invades deeper tissues.

Squamous Cell Carcinoma These tumours will more readily affect specific areas, such as areas exposed to ultraviolet, or the lips of smokers. It also affects some people who work with tar or heavy industrial oils. It is more commonly found in men over 45 years of age. The cells of the tumour resemble those of prickle cells, having fibrils which bridge the intercellular spaces. It is spread through the lymphatic system.

Malignant Melanoma This form of cancer usually only affects middle-aged and elderly people. About 50 per cent of cases may arise from existing moles. The mole, which may have been present for some time, may change colour or shape to become irregular both horizontally and vertically. It may become tender, itchy or even painful. Ulceration may develop at a later stage. Moles that have hair growing out of them are less likely to become cancerous.

Conditions Particularly Affecting Black Skin

Vitiligo This is the most well-known disorder. It is characterised by an absence of pigmentation. It may be a small area of discolouration or a full albinism.

Keloid Scarring Following injury, severe acne or surgery, the dermis produces a proliferation of cells, causing a raised area of dark, purplish tissue which can grow to be larger than the original scar tissue.

Hypersensitive Reaction Found in response to certain foods, chemical or protein substances, this is frequently found in black people. It may be manifest as puffy or odematous skin, or as a rash with skin irritability.

Disorders of the Sweat Glands

Hyperhidrosis The secretion of an excessive amount of sweat, which may have an offensive odour. It particularly affects the extremities, the axillae and the groin. It tends to be hereditary.

Anidrosis An absence of sweat, due to the destruction of sweat glands, or congenital factors.

Bromidrosis A condition in which the sweat has a particularly unpleasant odour. This is increased by bacterial decomposition.

Chapter 4

The Skeletal System

The whole skeleton consists of 206 bones. They can be classified according to shape.

Long bones. These consist of a shaft (diaphysis) and two broader ends (epiphysis). The *femur* is the longest bone in the body.

Short bones. These are similar in shape to long bones but have no shaft. The *carpals* (in the wrist) are short bones.

Flat bones. These include the *sternum* or breast bone.

Irregular bones. These include the *vertebrae.*

Sesamoid bones. These are rounded, such as the *patella* (knee).

The skull consists of 22 bones.

The skeletal system has six main functions:

1 The skeleton provides a framework, giving support for the rest of the body.
2 The system affords protection for vital organs.
3 The bones act as points of attachment for tendons and muscles.
4 The joints between bones allow mobility.
5 The system acts as a store for minerals such as calcium salts.
6 Blood cells are produced in the red bone marrow.

If bones were formed of solid masses, they would be too heavy for the rest of the body tissue to support or move (see Chapter 2). Some bones, like those of the face, have cavities in them called *sinuses* or antra. These help to make them lighter.

BONE TYPES

There are two types of bone: *cancellous bone* and *compact bone*.

Cancellous Bone

This has a spongy appearance rather like a honeycomb. It is formed by a criss-cross arrangement of bone tissue which gives it strength without too much

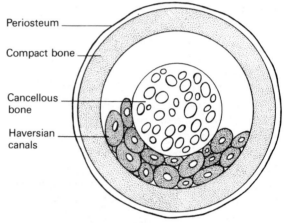

Periosteum

Compact bone

Cancellous bone

Haversian canals

Cross-section of a long bone

weight. Some examples are the sternum, ribs, clavicles and scapulae. The long bones of small children contain red bone marrow. As children get older, the red marrow recedes to the ends of the long bones to be replaced by yellow marrow containing fat cells. After the age of 25 years red marrow is only found in the sternum, ribs, clavicles and scapulae and the proximal ends of the humerus and femur. *Erythrocytes* (red blood cells) are formed in red bone marrow (see page 12).

Compact Bone

This surrounds cancellous bone. It is a hard substance rather like ivory, and is denser and less porous than cancellous bone. Compact bone gives a bone strength and rigidity as well as a smooth surface.

WITHIN THE BONE

Haversian Canals

These are very small circular canals in the bone, through which blood and lymph vessels pass in order to bring nourishment to these tissues (see page 12).

Periosteum

This is a thin membrane which covers all bones. It contains a rich supply of blood vessels and nerves and acts as an attachment for tendons.

BONE TISSUE

Bone tissue consists of approximately 25 per cent water, 30 per cent organic matter and 45 per cent minerals. The mineral content is mainly calcium phosphate with traces of magnesium salts, which helps to harden the bone tissue.

Bone cells, like all other cells, are constantly being replaced. The main bone-forming cells are called *osteoblasts*. They secrete collagen. This forms a matrix around the cell which is then called an *osteocyte*. Bones are eroded through the phagocytic action of *osteoclasts*.

JOINTS

A *joint* is where two or more bones meet, and is *a point of articulation*. Bones are held together by connective tissue called *cartilage*. There are three main groups of joints relating to the amount of movement they perform. They are:

diarthrosis (synovial) joints
amphiathrosis (cartilaginous) joints
synarthrosis (fibrous) joints.

Diarthrosis (Synovial) Joints

These are joints which usually have a considerable amount of movement between the bones. The joint is enveloped within a fine membranous capsule (sheath). This contains a viscous fluid called *synovial* fluid which acts as a lubricant between the two bones. The capsule is sometimes called a *bursa*. If it becomes inflamed, the condition is known as bursitis.

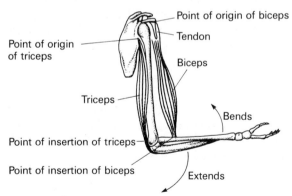

Point of origin of biceps
Tendon
Point of origin of triceps
Biceps
Triceps
Point of insertion of triceps
Point of insertion of biceps
Bends
Extends

A synovial joint

There are seven types of synovial joints, defined according to their type of action:

1 *Pivot*: where one bone turns on another (e.g. the radius and ulna at the elbow).
2 *Hinge*: which allows movement in one direction only (e.g. at the elbow).
3 *Double Hinge*: which allows movement in two directions (e.g. at the wrist).
4 *Gliding*: where bones glide over one another (e.g. at the wrist).
5 *Ball and Socket*: as, for example, where the hemispherical head of the femur fits into the cup-shaped socket to form the hip.
6 & 7 *Saddle and Condyloid*: where movement of one bone may take place at right angles to another (e.g. at the thumb).

Amphiathrosis (Cartilaginous) Joints

These have little or no movement depending on the amount of cartilage separating the bones, e.g. the joints of the vertebral column.

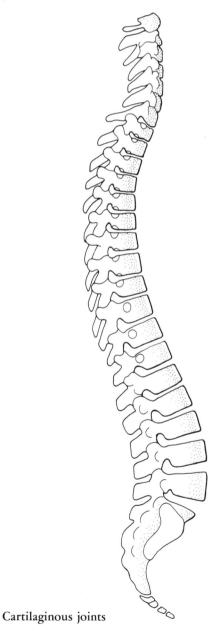

Cartilaginous joints

Synathrosis (Fibrous) Joints

There is virtually no movement between the bones of these joints. A strong, fibrous tissue bonds the bones together. Most of the bones of the skull fall into this category.

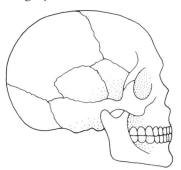

Fibrous joints

THE SKULL

The skull of an average adult weighs approximately 10 lbs ($4\frac{1}{2}$ kilos). It consists of 22 bones. Some are flat and some irregular. They fuse together in early infancy to form an immoveable casing. The only freely moveable bone is the mandible.

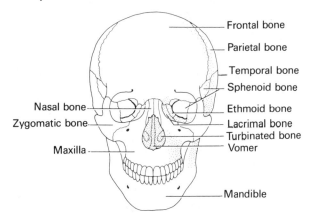

The skull: anterior view

The function of the skull is to protect the brain and to give form to the face. The bones of the skull are divided into two groups:

    the bones of the cranium
    the bones of the face.

The Bones of the Cranium

The cranium may be described as having two parts: the *base* upon which the brain rests, and the *vault* which surrounds and protects the brain and gives form to the shape of the head.

The eight bones forming the cranium are:

  1 frontal bone
  2 parietal bones
  2 temporal bones
  1 occipital bone
  1 sphenoid bone
  1 ethmoid bone.

The Frontal Bone

This is a broad, flat bone which gives form to the forehead, i.e. the front of the vault. A ridge marks the upper part of the eye socket along the brow line. Below this, the bone forms part of the orbital cavities.

The Parietal Bones

These are two flat bones which join together to form the main part of the vault of the cranium. They lie behind the frontal bone and above the temporal bones.

The Temporal Bones

These two bones lie on each side of the head below the parietal bones and in front of the occipital bone. They are flat bones, but also have irregular features. They are divided into four parts:

1 A flat fan-shaped area called the *squamous* part.
2 A thickened irregular part lying behind the ear called the *mastoid process*.
3 An irregular part protruding forward to form part of the zygomatic arch called the *zygomatic process*.
4 A part which forms part of the base of the skull and contains the organ of hearing called the *petrous* portion.

The Occipital Bone

This is a large, flat bone which joins the parietal to form the rear aspect of the vault and part of the base. It contains a large hole (*foramen magnum*) through which the spinal cord passes.

The Sphenoid Bone

This is an irregular-shaped bone which looks rather like an outstretched bat. It lies in the middle portion of the base. A saddle-shaped portion of it is called the *hypophyseal fossa*. It holds the pituitary gland. If there are abnormalities of this bone in the foetus, the baby may be born with deformities which include those affecting the bridge of the nose.

The Ethmoid Bone

This is an irregular-shaped bone lying at the front of the base. It forms part of the orbital cavities, the roof of the nose and the nasal septum.

The Bones of the Face

These bones either give form to the shape of the face or lie within the confines of the skull.

The thirteen bones of the face consist of:
- 1 mandible
- 1 maxilla (originally 2 bones: see below)
- 2 zygomatic bones
- 2 lacrimal bones
- 2 nasal bones
- 2 palatine bones
- 1 vomer
- 2 inferior conchae.

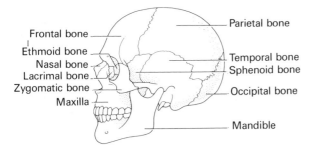

Frontal bone
Ethmoid bone
Nasal bone
Lacrimal bone
Zygomatic bone
Maxilla
Parietal bone
Temporal bone
Sphenoid bone
Occipital bone
Mandible

The skull: lateral view

The Mandible

This is the only moveable bone of the skull. It is formed by the fusion of the two bones at the mid-line which gives it strength. It articulates with the temporal bones. The curved body, lying horizontally, contains the lower set of teeth. The sides of the bone which project upwards are known as the *rami*. Where the ramus and the body join is known as the *angle of the jaw*.

The Maxilla

This irregular shaped bone is formed by the fusion of two bones during the first year of life. The front aspect contains the set of upper teeth. It also forms the front of the roof of the mouth, the floor of the nasal cavities and part of the orbital cavities.

The Zygomatic Bones

These two bones articulate with the zygomatic processes of the temporal bones. They form the prominence of the cheeks known as the *zygomatic arch*.

The Lacrimal Bones

These two bones form part of the inner aspect of the orbital cavities.

The Nasal Bones

These two small bones form the bridge of the nose.

The Palatine Bones

These irregular-shaped bones form part of the hard palate and the floor of the nasal cavities.

The Vomer

This is a thin, flat bone which forms part of the nasal septum.

The Inferior Conchae (Turbinated Bones)

These are shaped like a scroll and form part of the walls of the nasal cavities.

Cranial Bones

For the most part, the external surface of the cranium is smooth. The internal surface is uneven. It follows the surface of the brain and blood vessels which lie closely under it. The bones of the cranium vary in thickness according to where they lie.

Auditory Bones

Inside each ear are three small bones:
- 1 stapes bone (stirrup)
- 1 malleus bone (hammer)
- 1 incus bone (anvil).

Bones Close to the Skull

Hyoid Bone

This horseshoe-shaped bone lies in front of the trachea. It acts as an attachment for the tongue. It is often referred to as the 'Adam's Apple'. It is usually more prominent in men than in women.

THE SPINE

Thirty-three bones form the spine. Twenty-four of them are true vertebrae separated by cartilage pads. Nine are fused together and are known as *false vertebrae*.

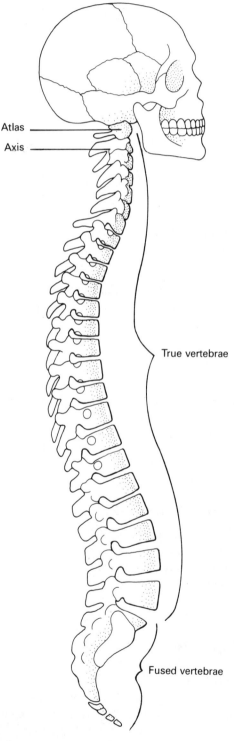

The spine

Seven cervical vertebrae form the neck. The top one is known as the *atlas* after the mythical character who supported the world upon his shoulders. The skull is tilted forward and backward on this bone. The second vertebra is known as the *axis*. The skull is rotated from side to side over this vertebra.

DISORDERS OF THE SKELETAL SYSTEM

Fracture This is the technical term for any broken bone. It can be caused by:

Direct Violence: when a bone is broken directly under the area where force was applied.

Indirect Violence: where the bone is fractured by a force applied at a distance from the site of the fracture and transmitted to the fracture site. For example, a clavicle can be fractured as a result of falling onto an outstretched hand.

Muscular Contraction: when the bone is broken by a sudden violent contraction of the muscles attached to it. For example: when the leg is twisted suddenly and the patella is fractured as a result of this.

There are three types of fracture:

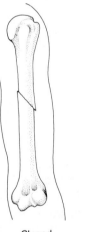 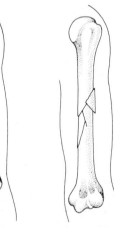

Closed   Open   Complicated

Types of fracture

Closed Fracture This is when a bone breaks in one place and there is no damage to the surrounding tissue.

Open Fracture This is when the bone has pierced the surrounding tissue and the skin.

Complicated Fracture This is where a broken bone has caused damage to other organs such as a large blood vessel, nerves or body organs.

Arthritis An inflammation of the joints.
Mono: affecting one joint.
Poly: affecting many joints.
Spondylitis: affecting the spine.
Osteo: affects hips, spine and hands particularly; produces swelling and loss of cartilage.
Rheumatoid: Firstly affects smaller, peripheral joints, and later also the larger joints. This may sometimes be due to a hormonal deficiency.

Periostitis Inflammation of periosteum.

Osteomyelitis Inflammation of a bone cavity.

Dislocation Where a bone is pulled out of position at a joint.

Synovitis Inflammation of the membrane lining of the cavity of a joint.

Bursitis Inflammation of a bursa.
Chronic: when fluid occurs in a bursal sac, e.g. housemaid's knee.
Acute: when an abscess occurs.

Gout A swelling and deformity of a joint caused by an excess of uric acid in the blood.

Chapter 5

The Muscular System

TYPES OF MUSCLE

There are over 640 named muscles in the body and many thousands of unnamed ones, such as the arrector pili muscles which make one's hair stand on end. Muscles make up about 45 per cent of the total body weight. They contain approximately 20 per cent water, 75 per cent protein, 5 per cent mineral salts, gases and a little fat.

Muscles receive nourishment in the form of oxygen, glycogen, glucose and lipids from the arterial blood supply. This is converted into energy by chemical changes. Waste products such as lactic acid and urea are removed from the muscles by the venous system. Particles that are too large for this system are collected by the lymphatic system.

Muscles are usually duplicated on each side of the body.

There are three types of muscle:

    voluntary muscles
    involuntary muscles
    cardiac muscles.

Voluntary Muscles (Skeletal, Striated)

These muscles are sometimes referred to as 'striped' muscles as they have regularly spaced bands of muscle fibres (see Chapter 2). The fibres are arranged in bundles of various sizes and in differing patterns.

Each bundle is contained in a sheath of fibrous tissue. Connective tissue lies between each bundle. A given pattern of bundles is enclosed in a stronger sheath of fibrous tissued called a *fascia*. These muscles are not uniform in their shape or size (see opposite).

Voluntary muscles usually move the skeletal frame. On the face they are often attached to other muscles or the skin, altering facial expression when moved. They are normally moved by a conscious effort from a motor nerve under stimulation from the brain.

Structure of a Voluntary Muscle

A muscle is composed of numerous elongated cells bound together and called fibres. These fibres are surrounded by a sheath called the *sarcolemma*. Bundles of these fibres lying in parallel fashion are known as *fasciculi*. These in turn are surrounded by a sheath of connective tissue called the *perimysium*. This sheath, as well as surrounding each fasciculus, is continuous with a tough fibrous sheath which covers the whole muscle. This outer sheath is called the *epimysium*. It extends to form the tendon by which the muscle is attached to other structures.

When muscles are stimulated by nerves they contract, that is, they become shorter. The main body of the muscle is called the *belly* of the muscle. Where a tendon is attached to a bone above a joint, this *fixed* point is called the *point of origin*. Where the tendon is attached below the joint, to the bone that is *to be moved*, this point is called the *point of insertion*.

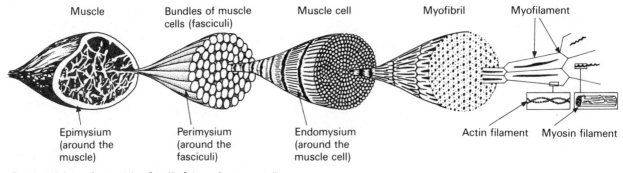

Muscle   Bundles of muscle cells (fasciculi)   Muscle cell   Myofibril   Myofilament

Epimysium (around the muscle)   Perimysium (around the fasciculi)   Endomysium (around the muscle cell)   Actin filament   Myosin filament

Cross-section of a muscle: detailed (see also page 14)

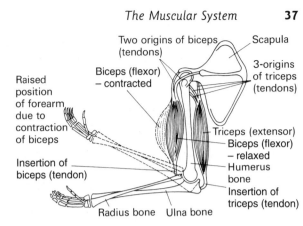

Antagonistic muscles of the forearm

Antagonistic muscles

Some muscles work in pairs: these pairs are called *antagonistic muscles*. These muscles are always under slight tension, as they act in opposite directions: when one is contracted, the other is relaxed. This state is called *muscle tone*. The muscle that performs the movement is called the *prime mover* (*synergist*). The muscle working to balance the prime mover is called the *antagonist*. When, for instance, the arm is flexed at the elbow, the biceps brachialis muscle in the upper arm is called into action. It has two points of origin, both arising at the proximal end of the humerus (i.e. near the shoulder) and one point of insertion, in the proximal end of the radius (just below the elbow). As the forearm is raised, the biceps shortens and becomes fatter in the belly (contracts).

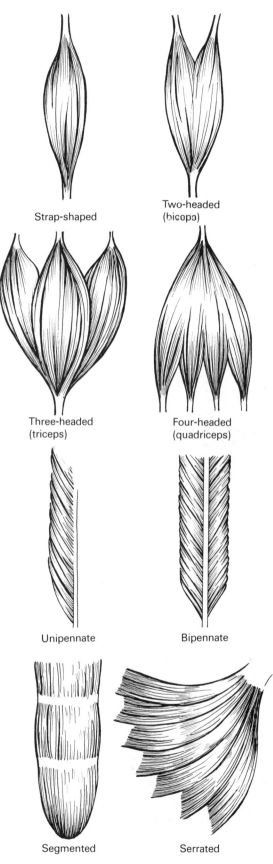

Strap-shaped

Two-headed (biceps)

Three-headed (triceps)

Four-headed (quadriceps)

Unipennate

Bipennate

Segmented

Serrated

Muscle shapes: voluntary muscles

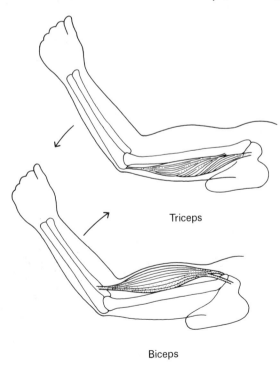

Triceps

Biceps

Extensor and flexor muscles

At the same time, the triceps lengthens and counter-balances it (relaxes). Thus the biceps acts as the prime mover, and the triceps as the antagonist.

Involuntary Muscles (Smooth, Non-striated)

These are a much simpler form of muscle and are rarely under direct voluntary control. They are normally part of the autonomic nervous system. However some muscles such as the diaphragm can be controlled for a short time, as when the breath is held. Involuntary muscles are found in the alimentary tract, blood and lymph vessels, the respiratory system and the skin.

Cardiac Muscles

These muscles are found only in the heart walls. They resemble voluntary muscles although the fibres are smaller. Their action is similar to involuntary muscles in that they are not under conscious control (see Chapter 7).

THE MAIN MUSCLES OF THE SKULL

These are often categorised as:

the muscles of the scalp
the muscles of facial expression
the muscles of mastication (of the nose and face).

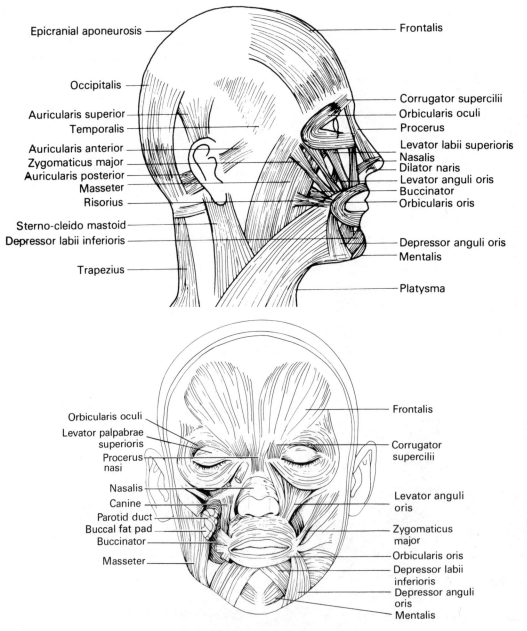

Main Muscles of the Skull

Name	Description	Origin	Insertion
MUSCLES OF THE SCALP			
Occipitofrontalis	The collective term for the occipital and frontalis muscles. They are normally used together but can be worked independently.		
Occipital	Covers the vault of the skull and occipital bone and draws the scalp backwards.	1 Occipital bone	1 Epicranial aponeurosis
Frontalis	Two muscles which usually act together. They cover the frontal bone, raise the eyebrows and draw the scalp forward. They also cause lines on the forehead. They are sometimes called the muscles of attention.	1 Epicranial aponeurosis	1 Skin under eyebrow
MUSCLES OF FACIAL EXPRESSION			
Eyes:			
Orbicularis Oculi	Circular sphincters which surround the eyes and close them. They relax when sleeping and can be used independently as when winking.	1 Medial part of orbital rim	1 Forms a sphincter around each eye and across the eyelids
Levator Palpebrae Superioris	Opens the eyelids and works as antagonist to the orbicularis oculi.	1 Back of the orbit	1 Upper eyelid
Corrugator Supercilii	Draws the eyebrows inwards and downwards causing the vertical lines on the forehead apparent when frowning.	1 Orbital arch	1 Skin under eyebrow
Nose:			
Procerus	Covers the top of the nose and wrinkles it, drawing the eyebrows inwards.	1 Fascia covering the lower part of nasal bone 2 Lateral nasal cartilage	1 Skin of lower part of forehead between eyes
Nasalis	Covers the tip of the nose and compresses it.	1 Maxilla	1 Bridge of nose
Depressor Septi	Lies above the upper lip. It elevates the side of the nose to widen the nasal aperture.	1 Maxilla	1 Upper lip
Dilator Naris: Posterior and Anterior	Lie inside the nasal cavities and dilate the nostrils.	1 Maxilla	1 Cartilaginous ala nasi
Mouth:			
Orbicularis Oris	A sphincter surrounding the mouth and closing the lips. It is known as the kissing muscle.	1 Sphincter around mouth	1 Into itself
Levator Labii Superioris	Lift the corners of the lips and assist in opening the mouth.	1 Maxilla 2 Zygomatic bone	1 Skin at angle of mouth 2 Upper lip
Depressor Labii Inferioris	Pull the corners of the mouth downwards. Assist in opening the mouth. Used together (both sides of the mouth) they can produce a dismal expression.	1 Platysma	1 Skin at angle of mouth 2 Lower lip
Levator Anguli Oris	Lying above the upper lip, they lift the corners of the mouth. Known as the muscles of threat.	1 Canine fossa of mandible	1 Other muscles at angle of mouth
Zygomaticus Major	Lift the corner of the mouth when laughing.	1 Zygomatic bone	1 Other muscles at angle of mouth
Zygomaticus Minor	Raise the upper lip, producing the mouth furrow. When used with other muscles they can express contempt.	1 Zygomatic bone	1 Upper lip
Mentalis	Covers the tip of the chin. It raises and causes the lower lip to protrude. Known as the muscle of disgust, it expresses doubt or disdain.	1 Mandible	1 Skin of chin

Name	Description	Origin	Insertion
Risorius	Lifts the corner of the mouth when smiling.	1 Parotid fascia	1 Skin at angle of mouth
Buccinator	Compress the cheeks in chewing or sucking. They are known as the whistling muscles.	1 Mandible 2 Maxilla	1 Muscles at angle of mouth
Ears (These muscles are very rudimentary in humans)			
Auricularis Anterior	Lying in front of the ears, they draw the ears forward.	1 Epicranial aponeurosis	1 The curve (helix) of ear
Auricularis Superior	Lying above the ears, they raise the ears slightly.	1 Epicranial aponeurosis	1 The flat (auricle) tendon of ear
Auricularis Posterior	Lying behind the ears, they draw them back slightly.	1 Epicranial aponeurosis 2 Temporal bone	1 Cartilage of ear auricle
MUSCLES OF MASTICATION **Face:**			
Temporalis	Shaped like a fan, they elevate the mandible to close the mouth. They also assist in side-to-side teeth grinding.	1 Temporal bone 2 Temporal fascia	1 Mandible 2 Mandible
Masseter	A broad muscle lying across the cheek. It raises the mandible in mastication and has a slight lateral movement used for grinding the teeth.	1 Maxilla 2 Zygomatic arch 3 Zygomatic arch	1 Angle of mandible 2 Mandible 3 Coronoid process of mandible
Lateral Pterygoid	Assists in opening the mouth by pulling the mandible forward.	1 Sphenoid bone 2 Pterygoid plate	1 Mandible 2 Temporo-mandibular disc
Medial Pterygoid	Elevates the mandible and helps to produce the side to side movement of the jaw.	1 Pterygoid plate 2 Maxilla 3 Palatine bone	1 Angle of mandible
MUSCLES OF THE NECK AND SHOULDERS			
Platysma	Lies at the front of the throat. Wrinkles the surface of the skin of the neck and assists in depressing the mandible. Draws down the lower lip at the angle of the mouth. It is seen in expressions of horror or surprise.	1 Fascia covering upper parts of pectoralis major and deltoid muscles	1 Mandible 2 Skin of lower part of face
Sternocleidomastoid	Lie at the front of the neck. If used separately, they turn the head from side to side. If used together, they flex the neck.	1 Sternum 2 Clavicle	1 Occipital bone 2 Temporal bone
Trapezius	Brace and raise the shoulders and extend the neck.	1 Occipital bone 2,3 Spines of cervical and thoracic vertebrae	1 Outer half of clavicle 2 Acromion process 3 Spine of scapula
Spinatus Erectae	Extend the vertebral column. Attached to the adjoining vertebra.		

DISORDERS OF THE MUSCULAR SYSTEM

Muscular Fatigue (specific or general) This is caused by over-exertion of muscles. It can lead to a build up of toxins in the area.

Fibrositis An inflammation of muscle fibres.

Rupture A tear across the muscle or muscle sheath resulting in a muscle hernia.

Sprain Over-use of a muscle or injury at a joint. It produces a rupture of the ligaments with severe bruising.

Cramp A spasmodic muscular contraction.
Swimmers: due to cold and exertion. It affects arteries as well as muscles.
Heat: particulary affects people who work in a very high temperature. They lose body salts through profuse sweating.
Writers: a spasm that can affect people performing repetitive movements, e.g. writing, sewing, telephonist work, etc.

Wry Neck A muscle spasm that draws the head to one side.

Chapter 6

The Neurological System

The Neurological (Nervous) System is of great importance to all the other body systems. It transmits messages to and from all the organs of the body. Part of it, the brain, acts as a store for information, rather like a computer.

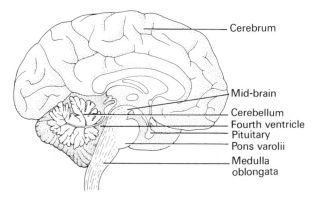

Section through the brain

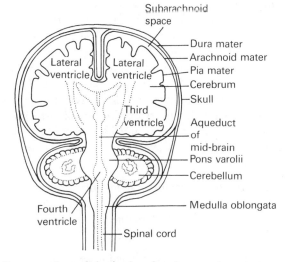

Cross-section of the brain, showing meninges

The neurological system is divided into two main parts, each with their own functions: the *central nervous system* and the *peripheral nervous system*.

Each system has both sensory and motor nerves.

THE CENTRAL NERVOUS SYSTEM

The central nervous system consists of the brain and the spinal cord. Because both of these are of such particular importance to the body, they are protected by bony cases: the bones of the skull and the spine. The brain and spinal cord are protected from being damaged by three strong membranes known as the *meninges*. They are individually called:

1 *The dura mater*. This has two layers and is the outer-most covering.
2 *The arachnoid mater*. The middle covering.
3 *The pia mater*. The innermost covering.

The Meninges

The outer and middle meninges are separated by what is called the *subdural space*. The arachnoid and pia maters are separated by the *subarachnoid space* which contains a clear, slightly alkaline fluid called *cerebrospinal fluid*. It is similar to blood plasma, but has added constitutents.

The functions of the meninges and cerebrospinal fluid are as follows:

1 They protect the brain and spinal cord through a cushioning effect against the surrounding bone.
2 They act to maintain a uniform pressure on the brain and spinal cord.
3 The outer layer of the dura mater takes the place of periosteum (which usually covers bone), lining the inner surface of the bones of the skull. The inner layer forms a loose sac around the brain. Outside the skull both layers fuse together to cover the spinal cord before fusing with the periosteum at the coccyx.
4 Both the arachnoid and pia maters closely follow the convolutions of the brain for added protection and a cushioning effect.

5 The pia mater contains a network of fine blood vessels.

6 The brain and spinal cord are kept moist, so avoiding a rubbing pressure.

7 The cerebrospinal fluid acts as a reservoir. The fluid can increase or decrease depending on the volume of the brain mass.

The Brain

The brain is the centre of the nervous system. It could be considered to be the most important part of the body. If it is severely damaged it may not fully recover. It receives and stores messages (impulses) in a retrievable system known as the *memory*. There are two types of memory: *short-term* and *long-term*. Long-term memory embraces the ability to remember aural or visual material; sensory experiences of taste, smell and touch; and concepts and ideas from the past; whether these have been experienced or learnt, either today or in our childhood.

The short-term memory carries information for a short period only. This could be just the time between looking up a telephone number and dialling it. The number is then forgotten.

A third type of memory is called *reflex* memory. This takes place mainly in the spinal cord and is an involuntary response to a stimulus. If an insect is felt walking on one's skin, the nervous reaction (reflex) is to brush it off. The long-term memory may then take over, remembering that the insect is a bee and that bees can sting.

The brain is formed from three main structures:

1 the *forebrain* consisting of:
   the cerebrum
   the thalamus
   the hypothalamus
2 the *brain stem* consisting of:
   the mid-brain
   the pons varolii
   the medulla oblongata
3 the *cerebellum* or hind-brain.

The Forebrain
THE CEREBRUM
This is the largest part of the brain. It is shaped rather like a walnut. The superficial surface of the cerebrum is known as the *cerebral cortex*. This is uneven, having folds known as *gyri* or *convolutions*, with depressions between them known as *sulci* or *fissures*. The purpose of the convolutions is to increase the surface area of the cerebral cortex.

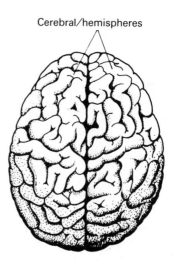

Cerebral/hemispheres

The cerebrum (dorsal view)

The cerebral cortex is composed of *grey matter*. This is made up of nerve cells which have no myelin sheath (non-myelinated). Lying under the grey matter is a mass of white cells. These are grey cells covered by short white fibres known as the myelin sheath (myelinated cells). (See pages 15–16.)

The cerebrum has a deep cleft called the *longitudinal cerebral fissure*. This divides the cerebrum into two parts called the right and left *cerebral hemispheres*. By a curious occurrence, the left hemisphere of the cerebrum governs the movement of the right side of the body. The right hemisphere is responsible for the movement of the left side of the body. This is known as *cerebral dominance*. A left-handed person is governed mostly by the right side of the cerebrum.

The cerebrum is associated with three main activities:

1 *Mental*: this includes memory, intelligence, the ability to reason, a sense of morality, learning and higher thought.
2 *Sensory*: this includes the concepts of temperature, touch, pain, sight, smell, taste and hearing.
3 *Conscious Control*: this governs the use of voluntary muscles.

Within each hemisphere lies a cavity filled with cerebrospinal fluid. These are called the right and left *lateral ventricles*. They communicate directly with another cavity called the *third ventricle*. This in turn communicates with the *fourth ventricle* which lies under the cerebellum.

Each hemisphere is divided into four *lobes*. They have the same names as the cranial bones under which they lie: frontal, parietal, temporal, occipital.

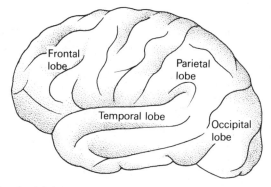

Cerebral lobes

1 The frontal and parietal lobes are separated by the central sulcus.
2 The temporal lobe is separated from the frontal and parietal lobes by the lateral sulcus.
3 The parietal and temporal lobes are separated from the occipital lobe by the parieto-occipital sulcus.

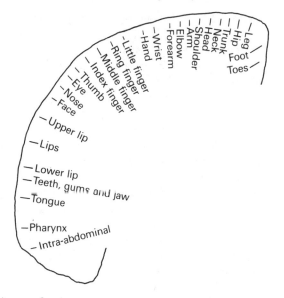

Areas of voluntary motor movements

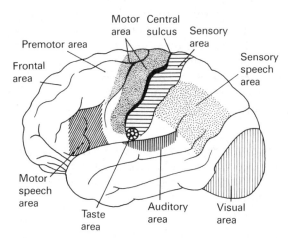

Association and motor areas of the brain

The Frontal Lobe Part of this is responsible for voluntary motor movements. Uppermost is the area responsible for the feet. Next is the area for the lower leg, then the knee and so on through the other parts of the body in ascending order. The area associated with speech is found in front of this motor area. It is governed by cerebral dominance. It is also thought to be responsible for behaviour, character, emotional traits and intellect.

The Parietal Lobe This is concerned with the sensations of heat, cold, touch, pain and limb position. It is thought to be the area responsible for remembering objects. The area for speech is also partly in this lobe.

The Temporal Lobe This is concerned with the senses of hearing, smell and taste, and also partly with speech.

The Occipital Lobe This is concerned with visual impulses and the sense of sight.

The two hemispheres of the cerebrum are linked to each other and to the different parts of the brain and spinal cord by both sensory and motor fibres. The bridge between the right and left hemispheres is called the *corpus callosum*. It is formed from masses of white nerve matter called *commissural fibre*. *Projection fibres* connect the cerebral cortex to the underlying grey matter and the spinal cord. *Association fibres* connect the different areas of the cerebral cortex within each hemisphere.

Lying deep within the cerebrum are masses of grey matter known as *ganglia*. They act as relay transmitters for stimuli. The *basal ganglia* is thought to influence skeletal muscle tone and muscle coordination. There are two important nerve relay centres in the forebrain: the *thalamus* and the *hypothalamus*.

THE THALAMUS
This is associated with sensory stimulations, relaying them to the specific area of the cerebral cortex.

THE HYPOTHALAMUS
This is an important part of the brain as it is linked to the pituitary gland.

The hypothalamus is responsible for the following:

1 Stimulating the pituitary gland to produce *oxytocin*, needed for lactation.
2 Stimulating the production of *vasopressin*, an anti-diuretic hormone required to concentrate urine.

3 Releasing hypothalamic hormones, which also act on the pituitary gland, persuading it to release either the *growth hormone* (GH) or the *growth hormone release inhibiting hormone* (GHRIH) which slows the growth rate.
4 Assisting in the regulation of body temperature.
5 Assisting in the control of appetite.
6 Assisting in the control of thirst.
7 Controlling the circadian rhythm so that the body has a natural rhythm of sleep, waking, and body functions.
8 Influencing sexual behaviour.
9 Stimulating emotional feelings and behaviour, such as fear and rage.
10 Affecting autonomic activities such as heart rate, vasomotor tone, and the secretory activity of the stomach and intestines.

The Brain Stem

The brain stem connects the cerebrum and cerebellum to the spinal cord. Several of the cranial nerves originate in the nerve cells of the medulla. It consists of: the *mid-brain*, the *pons varolii*, and the *medulla oblongata*.

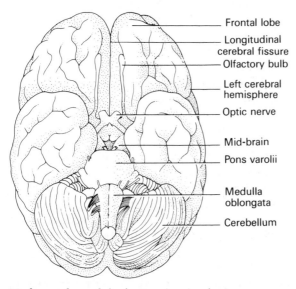

Frontal lobe
Longitudinal cerebral fissure
Olfactory bulb
Left cerebral hemisphere
Optic nerve
Mid-brain
Pons varolii
Medulla oblongata
Cerebellum

Under-surface of the brain: showing brain stem

THE MID-BRAIN

The mid-brain lies beneath the cerebrum and above the pons varolii. It acts as a relay station transmitting impulses along both ascending and descending nerve fibres. A particular function is to transmit impulses from the optical nerves. In so doing it plays a role in maintaining a sense of balance. It may also provide a reflex action of involuntary movement in response to a sudden loud noise or flash of bright light.

THE PONS VAROLII

The pons varolii lies in front of the cerebellum, below the mid-brain and above the medulla oblongata. It differs from the cerebrum in that the grey nerve cells lie deep in the structure, while the myelinated cells (fibres) lie on the surface (see page 42). These fibres act as a bridge between the two hemispheres of the cerebellum. The pons varolii acts mainly as a relay station for nerve impulses, especially those of the cranial nerves.

THE MEDULLA OBLONGATA

The medulla oblongata is situated below the pons varolii and is continuous with the spinal cord. It lies just above the foramen magnum (the hole in the skull where the brain stem joins the spinal cord). It is shaped rather like an inverted pyramid. Like the pons varolii, the grey nerve cells lie centrally with the white fibres surrounding them. On either side of the medulla lie two longitudinal swellings known as the *pyramids*. They contain the nerve fibres which link the cerebral cortex with the spinal cord. In the lower part of the medulla, most of these fibres cross over and pass down the opposite side of the spinal cord. This is how the right hemisphere has greater control of the left side of the body and vice versa. Where the crossover occurs is known as the *decussation of the pyramids*.

THE VITAL CENTRES

Within the grey matter lies the collections of cells associated with the autonomic reflex system called the vital centres. They are: the *cardiac centre*, the *respiratory centre*, the *vasomotor centre* and the *reflex centre*.

The Cardiac Centre

Within this, the sympathetic nerve fibres stimulate and so increase the rate and strength of the heart beat. The parasympathetic nerves' stimulation lowers the rate and the force of the heart beat.

The Respiratory Centre

This is stimulated either by an excess of carbon dioxide or a deficiency of oxygen in the blood. Nerve impulses pass to the phrenic and intercostal nerves. These in turn stimulate the diaphragm and intercostal muscles, so controlling the rate and depth of respiration.

The Vasomotor Centre

This stimulates the blood vessels, especially the small arteries and capillaries, through the autonomic nervous system. They may be dilated or constricted depending on the necessity for more or less blood in the site. The original stimulation may have been due to pain, fear, fainting or an emotional stimulus.

The Reflex Centre

This is responsible for the reflex actions associated with swallowing, coughing, sneezing or vomiting. It is stimulated by an irritation in the upper gastric or respiratory tracts.

THE RETICULAR FORMATION

Extending throughout the core of the brain stem is a network of grey cells interspersed with white nerve fibres. It is called the *reticular formation* and is part of the reticular activating system (RAS).

It acts rather like a telephone exchange receiving messages (impulses) from all parts of the nervous system in the body and directing them to the appropriate part of the brain. It also directs impulses, either directly or indirectly, back to all parts of the nervous system. Because of the vast number of impulses received, the reticular formation is involved particularly with the coordination of skeletal muscle activity and the maintenance of balance.

The reticular formation is also concerned with the hypothalamus and pituitary glands. It is associated with the autonomic systems of the cardiac, respiratory, vasomotor and reflex centres. It is also involved with sleep, arousal and the state of conscious alertness resulting from sensory impulses from all areas of the body.

The Cerebellum

The cerebellum lies behind the pons varolii, below the posterior part of the cerebrum. Like the cerebrum, it also has two hemispheres. The grey nerve cells form the surface and cover the white matter.

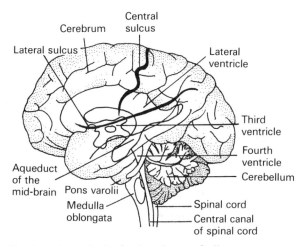

Section through the brain: the cerebellum

Three nerve tracts known as *cerebellar peduncles* allow the nerves of the cerebellum to connect with other parts of the brain.

Cerebellar activities are carried out at the subconscious level. They are concerned with coordination and the smoothness and precision of movement while it is happening. Impulses from the eyes and semicircular canals of the ears provide information about the position of the head and so influence the sense of balance.

The Spinal Cord

The spinal cord can be considered as part of the brain lying outside the skull. It is continuous with the medulla oblongata but lies within the vertebral column. It extends from above the first cervical vertebra to below the first lumbar vertebra. Like the brain, it is covered and protected by the meninges and cerebrospinal fluid. It gives off 31 pairs of spinal nerves which carry impulses to and from all parts of the body.

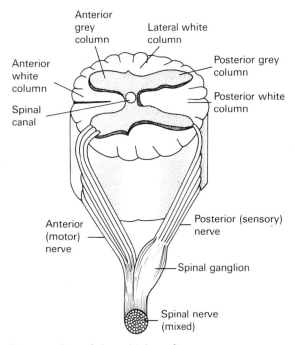

Cross-section of the spinal cord

A cross-section of the spinal cord shows a central canal containing cerebrospinal fluid. This is surrounded by an 'H' shape of grey matter. The projections are called *horns*. The two posterior horns convey sensory information. The two anterior horns carry motor information. At each side of the 'H' in the thoracic and lumbar parts of the spine is another projection, called the *lateral horn*. The grey matter also has *connector neurons* which link the sensory and the motor neurons together.

The whole of the 'H' structure is encased in an oval of white matter. In these white myelinated fibres there are three categories of nerve tract:

1 The sensory fibres, which convey impulses to the brain. They ascend in what are called the *posterior tracts*.
2 The motor fibres, which transmit messages from the brain, and form a tract at each side of the 'H' called the *pyramidal tract*.
3 Fibres of connective neurons. It is in these connector neurons that most of the reflex action takes place.

THE PERIPHERAL NERVOUS SYSTEM

The peripheral nervous system consists of:
    31 pairs of spinal nerves
    12 pairs of cranial nerves
    the autonomic nervous system.

The nerves of the peripheral nervous system are composed of:
Sensory (afferent) nerve fibres, which convey impulses from the receptor organs of the body to the spinal cord and the brain.
Motor (efferent) nerve fibres, which convey impulses from the brain to the effectors. These are the muscles and organs of the body which respond to stimuli from the brain.

Structure of a Nerve Pathway

Each nerve consists of numerous neurons (see pages 15–16). Sensory neurons have long dendrites and short axons. Motor neurons have longer axons and shorter dentrites.

In some neurons, the myelin sheath has spaces or breaks along its length. These are called the *nodes of Ranvier*. They assist in the rapid transmission of impulses along the nerve pathway. Those axons without this white matter are called *non-myelinated* neurons or *grey matter*. Between the axon terminal ends of one neuron and the ends of the dendrites of the next neuron is a 'space' known as the *synapse* (see page 16).

In the skin, sensory nerves start off as very fine branching sensory nerve endings (*tactile nerve endings*). They pick up the sensations of heat, cold, touch and pain. The motor nerves carrying impulses to the skeletal muscles end in fine branching filaments called *motor end plates*.

Impulses are transmitted along a nerve by a chemical action. When a nerve impulse is received at an axon it triggers the release of chemical transmitters such as *acetylcholine*. This stimulates the dendrites to accept the impulse (message). The chemical is then neutralised and the axon relaxes. Other chemical transmitters are believed to include noradrenalin, dopamine and 5 hydroxytryptamine.

Nerves do not always go directly from the brain to an area of the body. They sometimes branch and join nerve fibres from a different nerve to form a *plexus* or

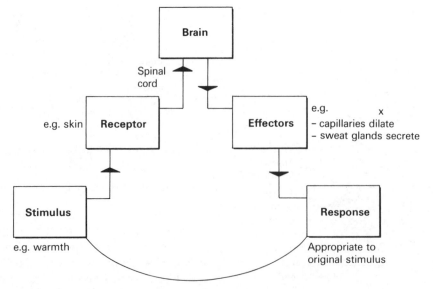

Sensory and motor stimulus pathway

network. There are five main plexus found on either side of the spinal cord: the *cervical*, the *brachial*, the *lumbar*, the *sacral* and the *coccygeal* plexus.

A nerve path does not consist of only one line of neurons. It is formed of numerous nerve fibres joined together in bundles. Like the brain, these bundles are well protected by several fine coverings.

Each nerve fibre is surrounded by *endoneurium*. Bundles of nerve fibres are surrounded by *perineurium*. Connective tissue called *epineurium* will protect several bundles of nerve fibres.

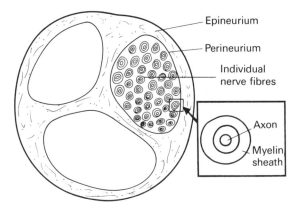

Bundles of nerve fibres

The Cranial Nerves

The brain gives off twelve pairs of cranial nerves which are associated with the different areas of the head and parts of the body. Some of them are sensory nerves, some of them are motor nerves, and some are bundles of both sensory and motor nerves and are called *mixed* nerves.

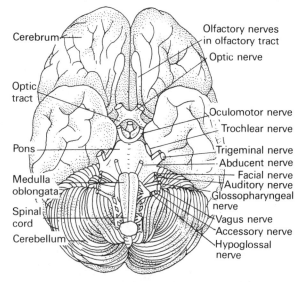

Inferior surface of the brain: showing cranial nerves

The Cranial Nerves

No.	Name	Type	Function
1	Olfactory	Sensory	Give a sense of smell. The nerve endings start in the mucous membranes in the upper part of the nose. They continue through the olfactory tract to the temporal lobe of the cerebrum.
2	Optic	Sensory	Convey a sense of sight. They begin in the retina of each eye. They pass through the back of the orbital cavity, through the optic coramin of the sphenoid bone. They join at the optic chiasma where the fibres from each eye cross over to go to the opposite side of the cerebrum.
3	Oculomotor	Motor	Supply the four main muscles that move the eyes: The superior, inferior, and medial recti; the inferior oblique muscles; the iris (which controls the amount of light permitted to enter the eye); the ciliary muscles.
4	Trochlear	Motor	Supply the superior oblique muscles, which move the eyes.
5	Trigeminal	Mixed	Sensory nerves: transmit the sensation of taste, heat and pressure. Motor nerves: stimulate the muscles of mastication. This is the largest of the cranial nerves. The trigeminal (3 pathway) nerve has three branches of sensory nerves: i) The ophthalmic branch transmits stimuli from the forehead and anterior aspect of the scalp; the upper eyelids; the lacrimal glands and the conjunctiva; and the mucous membranes lining the nose. ii) The maxillary branch transmits stimuli from the lower eyelids; the cheeks and side of the nose; the upper lip; gums and teeth. iii) The mandibular branch transmits stimuli from the side of the scalp and cheeks, including the upper part of the ear pinna; the chin and the lower lip; gums and teeth; and the tongue.
6	Abducent	Motor	Supply the lateral rectus muscles which move the eyeballs.
7	Facial	Mixed	Sensory nerves: transmit impulses from the taste buds in the anterior two-thirds of the tongue. Motor nerves: convey impulses to the muscles of facial expression.

8	Auditory	Sensory	There are two branches:
			i) The vestibular branch conveys impulses from the semicircular canals in the inner ear to the cerebellum. It therefore affects the sense of balance and equilibrium.
			ii) The cochlea branch transmits impulses from the inner ear to the cerebral cortex where they are perceived as sound.
9	Glossopharyngeal	Mixed	Sensory nerves: transmit impulses from the tonsils, pharynx and the taste buds in the posterior third of the tongue to the medulla oblongata. Motor nerves: stimulate the muscles of the pharynx and the secretory (saliva) cells of the parotid glands.
10	Vagus	Mixed	This nerve has the largest distribution area of the cranial nerves. Sensory nerves: transmit impulses from the membranes of the heart; blood vessels of the thorax and abdomen; the pharynx, larynx, trachea, oesophagus, stomach, intestines, pancreas, spleen, gall bladder, bile ducts, kidneys and ureters to the medulla oblongata. Motor nerves: supply the smooth muscles and secretory glands of the same organs.
11	Accessory	Motor	Supply the sternocleidomastoid and trapezius muscles which move the head and shoulders. It also supplies the muscles of the pharynx and larynx.
12	Hypoglossal	Motor	Supply the muscles of the tongue enabling it to move, and also the muscles surrounding the hyoid bone in the front of the throat.

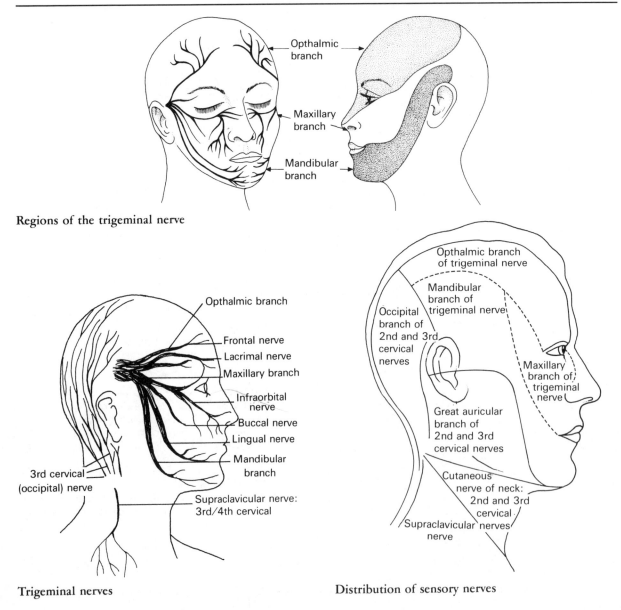

Regions of the trigeminal nerve

Trigeminal nerves

Distribution of sensory nerves

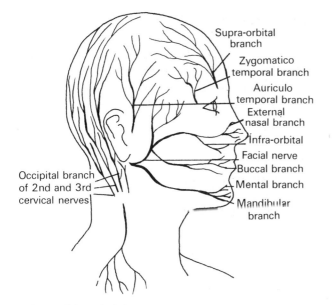

7th cranial or facial nerve

Labels on diagram:
- Supra-orbital branch
- Zygomatico temporal branch
- Auriculo temporal branch
- External nasal branch
- Infra-orbital
- Facial nerve
- Buccal branch
- Mental branch
- Mandibular branch
- Occipital branch of 2nd and 3rd cervical nerves

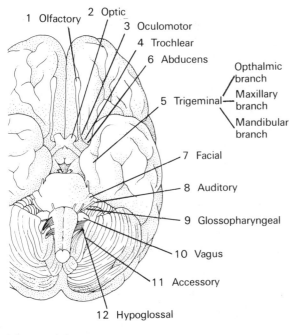

The cranial nerves

Labels on diagram:
- 1 Olfactory
- 2 Optic
- 3 Oculomotor
- 4 Trochlear
- 6 Abducens
- 5 Trigeminal — Opthalmic branch, Maxillary branch, Mandibular branch
- 7 Facial
- 8 Auditory
- 9 Glossopharyngeal
- 10 Vagus
- 11 Accessory
- 12 Hypoglossal

THE AUTONOMIC NERVOUS SYSTEM

The word *autonomic* means 'self control'. Therefore the autonomic nervous system is concerned with the involuntary functions that take place within the body. This could be an action such as the opening and closing of the heart's valves so as to produce a regular heart beat. Some people, such as athletes, have learnt

how to control their bodies so that they do not increase their heart rate on exertion as much as non-athletes.

The autonomic nervous system consists of two sets of nerves: the *sympathetic* and the *parasympathetic*. They act antagonistically or in opposition to each other. This forms a balance in the regulating of the organs and glands in the body.

The Sympathetic Nervous System

The sympathetic nerves increase and speed-up body activity. The motor sympathetic nerves originate in the nerve cells of the brain. They emerge from between the mid-brain and the sacral vertebrae. They then often pass along the same pathway as the peripheral nerves.

In order for the sympathetic nervous system to be distributed to all parts of the body it has to pass through the two *sympathetic trunks*. These lie on either side of the spinal column. They are each made up of a chain of sympathetic ganglia. The *preganglionic* nerves coming from the spinal cord may join, or synapse, with the sympathetic trunk at the same level. However, some may pass up or down the trunk to synapse at another ganglion.

The sympathetic nerves of the head either originate from the first thoracic vertebra via the sympathetic trunk or from the 9th, 10th, 11th or 12th cranial nerves. These are the ones that supply the ciliary muscles of the eyes, the blood vessels of the head, the salivary glands, and the oral and nasal mucosa. The action of the sympathetic nerves on these organs is to dilate the pupils of the eyes, constrict the bloodflow to the head and inhibit secretion from the salivary glands and oral and nasal mucosa. In the body, the sympathetic nerves increase the heart rate and reduce peristalsis in the stomach.

The sympathetic nervous system increases the action of sweat glands in the skin, resulting in heat loss and so regulating body temperature. Because the parasympathetic nervous system does not supply the skin, the sympathetic nervous system has a dual role there. It can both dilate and constrict the blood vessels, so is also able to prevent heat loss. It also contracts the arrector pili in the skin, raising the hairs and causing 'goosepimples'.

Sympathetic neurons secrete *noradrenaline*. This helps the body to deal with excitement and stress, preparing it to 'fight or take flight' from a situation.

The Parasympathetic Nervous System

The parasympathetic nervous system acts as the peace-keeper, helping the body to keep calm. This is because the parasympathetic neurons secrete *acetyl-choline*. Unlike the sympathetic nervous system, only a few of the parasympathetic nerves are given off directly from the spinal cord from the 2nd, 3rd and 4th lumbar vertebral junctions. The main parasympathetic nerves are, however, part of the cranial nervous system:

Nerve 3 (oculomotor) – this constricts the pupils of the eyes.

Nerve 7 (facial) – this increases saliva secretions and tears.

Nerve 9 (glossopharyngeal) – this also increases saliva.

Nerve 10 (vagus) – this is the most important nerve as it acts on most of the internal organs. Its functions include decreasing the heart rate and increasing the gastric juices.

The facial muscles and skin are supplied by superficial nerves mainly from the 5th (trigeminal) and 7th (facial) cranial nerves.

Muscles are moved by contraction. These are caused by nerve impulses. Small muscles usually only have a single nerve supplying them. Larger body muscles may be stimulated by more than one nerve. The point where the muscle receives the greatest amount of stimulation is called a *motor point*.

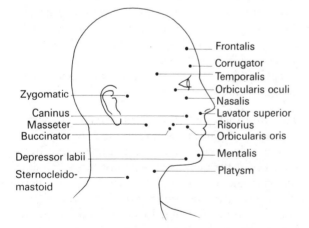

Motor points of the head

For details of the nerves of the hands and feet, see Chapter 8.

ORGANS OF SPECIAL SENSES

Sensation may be experienced in several ways: through sight, sound, taste, smell and touch. It involves the organs of the eyes, ears, tongue, nose and the skin. (For details of the skin, see Chapter 3.)

The Eyes

The eyes are the organs responsible for transmitting the images of vision to the *optic* (2nd cranial) nerve and thence to the brain for recognition. They lie in the *orbital cavities* formed by the frontal, sphenoid, ethmoid and lacrimal bones and are protected by connective tissue and fat.

The eyeballs are spherical in shape. Their walls are made up of three layers. These are: the *sclera*, the *choroid* and the *retina*.

The *iris* is the coloured part of the eye. The black circular area in its centre is called the *pupil*. The iris dilates or contracts to control the amount of light entering the eye. The eye can move in all directions, using its six muscles.

The four straight muscles are:
The superior rectus – which rotates the eyeball upwards.
The inferior rectus – which rotates the eyeball downwards.
The medial rectus – which rotates the eyeball inwards.
The lateral rectus – which rotates the eyeball outwards.

The two oblique muscles are:
The superior oblique – which turns the eyeball downwards and outwards.
The inferior oblique – which turns the eyeball upwards and outwards.

The eye contains:

1 The *lens*, a bi-convex body lying behind the iris. This helps to focus images on to the optic nerve.
2 *Aqueous humour*, a watery fluid that fills the anterior chamber between the lens and the cornea.
3 *Vitreous humour*, a jelly-like substance that fills the posterior chamber behind the lens.

The front of the eyeball is protected by an *eyelid* which helps to keep out the light, and *eyelashes* to keep out dust and other foreign matter. These have a number of small sebaceous and sweat glands. If one of these glands becomes infected it gives rise to a condition known as a *stye*. The eyelids are lined with a layer of mucous membrane called *conjunctiva*. An infection of this is called *conjunctivitis* or *pink eye*.

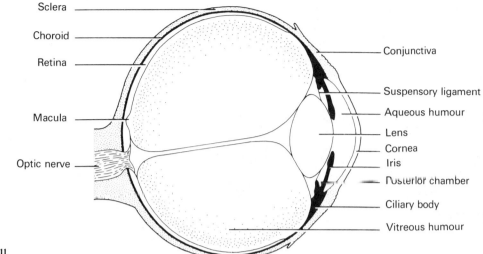

Sclera
Choroid
Retina
Macula
Optic nerve

Conjunctiva
Suspensory ligament
Aqueous humour
Lens
Cornea
Iris
Posterior chamber
Ciliary body
Vitreous humour

The eyeball

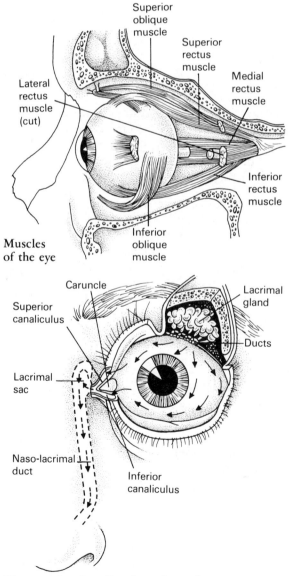

Superior oblique muscle
Superior rectus muscle
Medial rectus muscle
Lateral rectus muscle (cut)
Inferior rectus muscle
Inferior oblique muscle

Muscles of the eye

Caruncle
Superior canaliculus
Lacrimal gland
Ducts
Lacrimal sac
Naso-lacrimal duct
Inferior canaliculus

The eye: showing direction of tear flow

The eye is kept clear by being constantly washed by *lacrimal fluid* secreted by the *lacrimal gland*. These glands lie above the eye. The tears wash across the eye and into a small canal which leads into the nasal duct. If the eyes are not kept moist, they become dry and painful and there is a danger of them being scratched by dirt or grit.

The Ear

The ears are part of the organs which pick up sound and convey it to the brain. They are supplied by the *auditory* (8th cranial) nerve.

The ear can be divided into:

the external ear
the middle ear
the inner ear.

The External Ear

This is a form of cartilage covered with skin. Its function is to 'catch' sound and channel it down to:

The Middle Ear

This is a cavity which contains three small, connected bones: the *malleus*, *incus* and *stapes*. Air pressure within the middle ear is equalised through a narrow tube called the *eustachian tube*, which leads from the middle ear to the nasal part of the pharynx: the nasopharynx. The three auditory bones oscillate and conduct sound to:

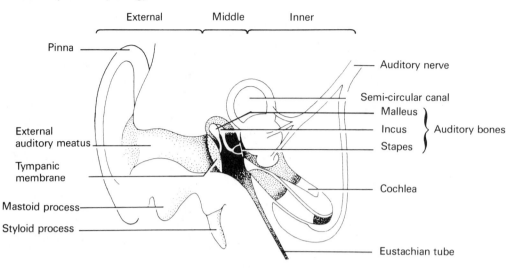

External   Middle   Inner

Pinna

Auditory nerve

Semi-circular canal

Malleus
Incus   } Auditory bones
Stapes

External
auditory meatus

Tympanic
membrane

Cochlea

Mastoid process

Styloid process

Eustachian tube

The ear

The Inner Ear

This consists of three *semicircular canals* which help to control balance, and the *cochlea* which is a narrow tube filled with fluid and numerous nerve endings. This translates the vibrations of the auditory bones into nerve impulses through the nerve endings, which terminate in the auditory nerve; which transmits sound to the brain.

The most common disorder of the ear is caused by too much wax or other foreign bodies being pushed into the ear.

The Tongue

The tongue is the organ of taste. It also assists in the process of breaking down food, swallowing and speech. It is supplied by the 7th (facial) and 9th (glossopharyngeal) cranial nerves. It is also supplied by the motor nerves of the 12th (hypoglossal) cranial nerves.

The tongue is covered with *papillae*. Within the papillae are numerous taste buds. These are the end pads of the 7th and 8th cranial nerves.

The taste buds do not all respond to the same sort of sensations. The tip of the tongue responds to the taste of sweet and salty flavours. It is also very sensitive to touch, pressure, pain and temperature. The sides of the tongue respond to sour flavours, while the back of the tongue senses bitter flavours.

The Nose

The nose is the sensory organ of smell. It also forms part of the respiratory system. The sensory nerve endings are found in the mucous membranes lining the roof of the nose. The sensation is carried by the 1st (olfactory) cranial nerve.

Human beings are generally less sensitive to odours than other animals. The sense of smell can be diminished by constantly being subjected to a particular odour, or by inflammation of the mucous membranes (as when one has a cold).

The sense of smell is important in that it can give warning of such things as contaminated food or an escape of gas.

DISORDERS OF THE NERVOUS SYSTEM

Damage to Nerves If a motor nerve is damaged, it can sometimes regenerate along its original path. Sometimes a sensory nerve will take over its function. Where nerves are damaged by alcohol or drugs, the motor nerve may convey altered or hallucinatory messages to the brain.

Bell's Palsy The 7th (facial) cranial nerve is affected. It causes pain and partial paralysis of one or both sides of the face. It may be caused by a draught, tooth decay or a blow to the head.

Herpes Zoster (Shingles) This is caused by a virus similar to chicken pox attacking nerve ganglia. The spinal nerves of the chest and the 5th cranial nerve are those most often affected. It may cause severe neuralgia or neuritis.

Neuralgia Pain along a nerve pathway.

Neuritis Inflammation of a nerve.

Parkinson's Disease A degeneration of nerve cells (grey matter) lying at the base of the brain. It causes a deficiency of the neurotransmitter *dopamine*. This results in a lack of muscle coordination which may cause trembling, rigid limbs and a mask-like face.

Sclerosis A hardening of an organ.

Multiple Sclerosis Hardened patches varying in size from a pinhead to a pea found through the brain and spinal cord. It is a progressive disease of unknown origin. At the onset there are tremors and temporary paralysis. Later the limbs become rigid.

Poliomyelitis This is caused by a virus which attacks the motor cells in the anterior horn of the spinal cord. The cranial nerves and certain cells in the brain may also be affected. The limbs may become weakened or paralysed. In severe cases the diaphragm and muscles of respiration may be involved.

Chapter 7

The Cardio-vascular and Lymphatic Systems

The cardio-vascular system consists of the heart, the blood vessels and the blood.

THE HEART

The heart is the pump that enables blood (containing oxygen and nutrients) to course through the blood vessels to all the other organs of the body.

The heart is a hollow, cone-shaped muscular organ. It is roughly the size of its owner's fist, weighing approximately 250 grams (9 ounces) in the female adult. The male heart is a little larger and heavier.

It lies just behind and a little to the left of the sternum. The *apex* of the cone points downwards and towards the left, at the level of the fifth intercostal space (i.e. just below the nipple line – slightly nearer to the midline). The *base* of the cone lies just below the level of the second rib.

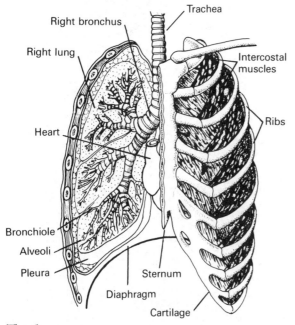

The thorax

The heart is formed from three layers of tissue:

    the pericardium
    the myocardium
    the endocardium.

The Pericardium

The pericardium is the outer covering of the heart. It is made up of two sacs. The outer layer is called the *parietal pericardium*. It is made of fibrous tissue and prevents distension of the heart. The parietal pericardium anchors the heart to the central tendon of the diaphragm, the sternum and the major blood-vessels, so that it does not move freely within the thorax.

The inner sac is called the *visceral pericardium*. It is attached to the underlying heart muscle. It is formed from serous membrane comprised of flattened epithelial cells. A serous fluid is secreted into a space called the *potential space*. This is to prevent the sacs rubbing against one another.

The Myocardium

This layer is formed from a special muscle tissue (see Chapter 2). It is thickest at the base of the heart and becomes thinner at the apex. The muscle tissue on the left side of the heart is thicker than on the right because it performs more work.

The Endocardium

This is a smooth, fine membrane formed from squamous epithelial cells. It is continuous with the lining of the blood vessels.

Structure of the Heart

The heart is divided into two halves by a strong muscular tissue called the *septum*.

Each side of the heart is divided into two chambers. The upper chambers are called *atria* (singular 'atrium'). The lower chambers are called *ventricles*. The atria are separated from the ventricles by strong, one-way valves formed from endocardium and fibrous tissue. The valves are prevented from opening the wrong way by ligaments called *chordae tendineae*. These are held in place by muscular projections in the walls of the ventricles. The valve separating the right atrium from the right ventricle has three flaps or cusps. It is called the *tricuspid* valve. The valve separating the left atrium from the left ventricle has only two flaps or cusps. It is called the *mitral* or *bicuspid* valve. The purpose of the valves is to stop blood from flowing backwards into the heart.

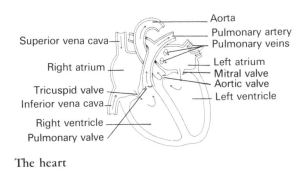

The heart

Bloodflow through the Heart

Blood enters the heart via the *superior* and *inferior venae cavae*. These are the largest veins in the body. They pour their contents into the right atrium. The atrium contracts and the blood passes through the tricuspid valve into the right ventricle. The pressure of blood inside the ventricle is higher than in the atrium. This puts pressure on the underside of the tricuspid valve so preventing a backflow of blood. The muscles of the atrium then relax so that it again fills with blood. At the same time, the muscles of the ventricle contract, pushing the blood through the *pulmonary* valve (formed from three semilunar cusps) into the two *pulmonary arteries*. These are the only arteries to carry deoxygenated blood. The blood then travels to the lungs. The right ventricle then relaxes.

Oxygenated blood enters the left atrium from the lungs via the four pulmonary veins. The muscles of the atrium contract (*atrial systole*) and the blood is pushed through the mitral valve into the left ventricle; then the muscles of the atrium relax. The muscles of the left ventricle then contract (*ventricular systole*) and the blood is pumped through the three semilunar cusps forming the *aorta valve* into the *aorta* (artery). Following the ventricular systole there is a period of rest for both atria and ventricles called the *diastole*. The cycles are then repeated.

Both atria are filled and relaxed at the same time. The ventricles are also filled and relaxed together.

Conducting System of the Heart

All muscular activity is in response to nervous stimulation. Situated near the opening of the superior vena cava lies a mass of specialist cells called the *sino-atrial node* (SA node). It is known as a *cardiac pacemaker* because it is able to generate impulses which cause the atria to contract, determining rate of heart beat. It also stimulates the atrioventricular node (AV node), which lies near the mitral valve.

Leading from the AV node in the septum are bundles of fibres called the *bundles of His*. They branch to follow the outline of the ventricles and form a fine network called the *fibres of Purkinje*. The impulses from the atrioventricular node cause the cardiac muscle at the apex of the heart to go into a wave-like contraction. This pushes the blood up into the pulmonary artery and the aorta. Both the SA node and the AV node are able to initiate stimulation of cardiac muscle impulses.

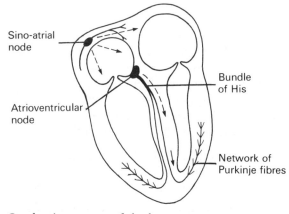

Conducting system of the heart

The heart is under the control of the autonomic nervous system. The parasympathetic part of the vagus (10th cranial) nerve has the effect of decreasing both the speed of the heart rate and the force of the heart beat. The sympathetic nerves have the reverse effect. The heart rate and strength is usually increased at times of exercise or excitement and decreased while the body is at rest.

Blood Pressure

The pressure that blood exerts within the blood vessels is known as *blood pressure*. Pressure is higher in arteries than in veins. When the left ventricle contracts it pumps blood into the aorta, which is already full. The aorta expands slightly to accommodate this extra blood. The blood is now under maximal arterial pressure; this is called *systolic blood pressure*. It is measured in millimetres of mercury. In the adult it registers approximately 120 mm Hg. In the diastolic period (ventricular diastole) when the heart is resting, there is minimal arterial pressure; this is called *diastolic blood pressure*. It registers 80 mm Hg. Blood pressure is measured by an instrument called a *sphygmomanometer*. The measurement is usually shown thus:

$$BP = \frac{120}{80} \text{ mm Hg}$$

THE BLOOD VESSELS

Blood vessels are responsible for carrying blood all over the body, to and from the heart. The three main categories are:

arteries
veins
capillaries.

The Arteries

These are the vessels which carry oxygenated blood from the heart to the capillaries in all the organs of the body. The smallest branches given off by the arteries are called *arterioles*. Although they vary in size, arteries all consist of three layers of tissue: tunica adventitia, tunica media and tunica intima.

Tunica Adventitia This is the outermost layer. It consists of collagen and elastic fibrous tissue. This gives both strength and protection to the vessel.

Tunica Media This is the middle layer. It consists of yellow elastic fibres in smooth muscle fibre.

Tunica Intima This is the innermost layer. It is formed from a layer of flattened endothelial cells lying over a layer of elastic fibres.

The larger arteries have proportionately more elastic tissue than the smaller arteries; while the smaller arteries have more muscle tissue. The arterioles (small arteries) consist mainly of smooth muscle tissue. The arterial muscles help to pump the blood

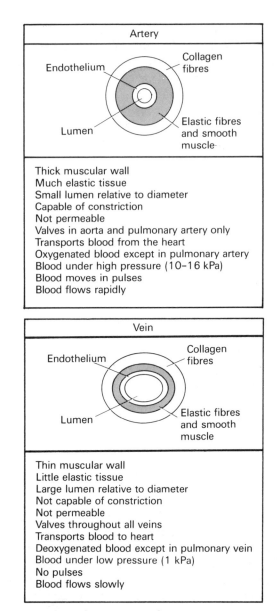

Thick muscular wall
Much elastic tissue
Small lumen relative to diameter
Capable of constriction
Not permeable
Valves in aorta and pulmonary artery only
Transports blood from the heart
Oxygenated blood except in pulmonary artery
Blood under high pressure (10–16 kPa)
Blood moves in pulses
Blood flows rapidly

Thin muscular wall
Little elastic tissue
Large lumen relative to diameter
Not capable of constriction
Not permeable
Valves throughout all veins
Transports blood to heart
Deoxygenated blood except in pulmonary vein
Blood under low pressure (1 kPa)
No pulses
Blood flows slowly

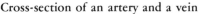

Cross-section of an artery and a vein

around the body. They do this by expanding as blood is pumped from the heart, and then contracting as the blood passes along the artery.

The Veins

Veins carry deoxygenated blood from all organs of the body back to the heart. Veins also have three layers of tissue, corresponding to those in the arteries. These are, however, much finer and contain less elastic fibres. Unlike the arteries, many veins have *valves* within them. Blood in the veins is not pumped around the body as is arterial blood. Pressure from organs other than the heart assists in the blood flow back to the heart. The valves stop the blood from stagnation or even flowing backwards.

Some of the veins are called *deep veins*: they follow the pathways of arteries. Others are called *superficial veins*: these are found near the surface of the body. The very smallest veins are called *venules*.

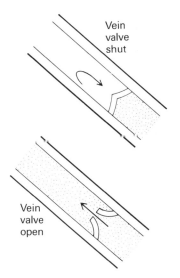

Veins: showing valves

Capillaries

These are very small blood vessels which branch from the arterioles. They are found throughout the tissues of the body. Capillaries consist of a single, loose layer of epithelial cells. There are spaces within this layer to allow white blood cells to move into and out of the surrounding tissue. This is so that oxygen and nutrients may be transported to the tissues, and carbon dioxide and other waste products removed. Capillaries then drain into venules (small veins) to carry the blood back to the heart.

THE CIRCULATORY SYSTEM

The circulatory system may be considered as three separate systems. They are:

    the systemic or general circulatory system
    the pulmonary system
    the portal system.

The Systemic or General Circulatory System

Blood leaves the left ventricle of the heart, passing into the aorta. This passes upwards to become the *ascending aorta*. It then forms the *arch of the aorta*, passing backwards and to the left before becoming the *descending aorta*. From here, many arteries are

given off going to the organs of the thorax, abdomen and limbs.

Leading off from the ascending aorta are the right and left *coronary arteries*. They carry blood and nutrients to the tissues of the heart itself.

Given off from the arch of the aorta are three arteries: the brachiocephalic artery, the left common carotid artery and the left subclavian artery.

Arterial Blood Supply to the Head

The *brachiocephalic artery* branches to form the *right common carotid artery* and the *right subclavian artery*.

The two common carotid arteries pass up the sides of the neck and then divide to become the external and internal carotid arteries.

The right and left external carotid arteries divide to give off four main branches: the facial artery, the occipital artery, the superficial temporal artery and the maxillary artery.

The *superior thyroid* and *lingual* arteries are given off at the side of the throat.

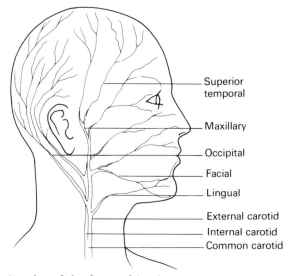

Arteries of the face and head

The internal carotid artery divides to form four main arteries: the ophthalmic artery, the anterior cerebral artery, the middle cerebral artery and the posterior communicating artery.

The *ophthalmic artery* supplies the eye.

The *anterior* and *middle cerebral arteries* and the *posterior communicating arteries* supply the different areas of the brain. They join together and, with the *anterior communicating arteries*, form the *circulus arteriosus* (circle of Willis) at the base of the brain.

Venous Blood Return from the Head

Blood is returned to the heart by a network of deep and superficial veins. They often have the same name as the corresponding arteries.

Within the dura mata covering of the brain are five *venous sinuses* where blood may be collected. They are:

1 superior sagittal sinus
1 inferior sagittal sinus
1 straight sinus
2 transverse sinuses.

The main veins join together with smaller superficial veins draining the face to form the *external jugular vein*. This, together with the *internal jugular vein*, forms the right and left *brachiocephalic veins*. These pass down the sides of the neck to join the *subclavian vein* from the arms. The two brachiocephalic veins join to form the *superior vena cava*. This drains blood into the right atrium of the heart.

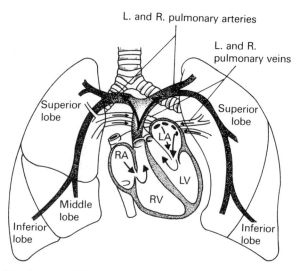

The heart and lungs

lung has three lobes. The left lung has only two lobes. Each lung contains air passages called *bronchi*. These branch into tiny *bronchioles* which further divide into minute *alveoli*. The arteries keep on dividing to become arterioles. They finally end in a dense network of capillaries which connect with the alveoli.

The arterial capillaries discharge their deoxygenated gasses and take in oxygen. The exchange takes place across fine membranes between the alveoli and capillaries.

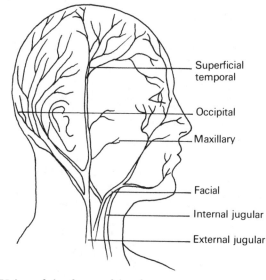

Veins of the face and head

The Pulmonary System

This is the circulation system whereby deoxygenated blood is taken from the heart to the lungs and returned carrying oxygen.

The deoxygenated blood leaves the right ventricle of the heart via the *pulmonary artery*. This is the only artery to carry deoxygenated blood. All the other arteries carry blood containing oxygen. The pulmonary artery divides into the right pulmonary artery and the left pulmonary artery.

The branches pass to the *superior lobes* of the right and left lungs. They divide into two further branches, passing to the other lobes of the lungs. The right

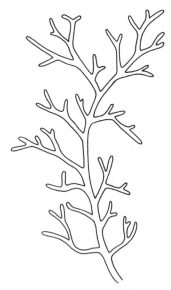

Capillaries

The venous capillaries leaving the alveoli then become venules. These become four pulmonary veins, two from each lung. They pour the oxygenated blood into the left atrium of the heart. They are the only veins to carry oxygenated blood.

The Portal System

The portal system is concerned with the blood supply to the intestines, the spleen and the liver.

BLOOD

Blood is considered to be part of the connective tissue of the body. It is a liquid and is always being transported from one organ to another. It carries nutrients, oxygen and hormonal outpourings to the tissues and transports waste matter to other organs to be excreted.

There are between eight and ten pints (5–6 litres) of blood in the adult, weighing about $\frac{1}{20}$ of the total body weight.

Blood is composed of:

  plasma
  erythrocytes (red blood corpuscles)
  leucocytes (white blood cells)
  platelets.

Plasma

Plasma is a clear, straw-coloured fluid. The blood cells are suspended in it. Plasma is a slightly alkaline fluid containing:

  Water: 90%
  Proteins: 60 g/l including:
    albumin 35–50 g/l
    globulin 20–39 g/l
    prothrombin 100–150 mg/l
    fibrinogen 2–4 g/l
  Minerals: (Inorganic) salts such as chlorides, sulphates, phosphates of sodium, potassium, calcium, magnesium, iron, copper, iodine
  Nutrients: such as amino acids, glucose (monosaccharides), fatty acids, glycerol, vitamins
  Gases: such as oxygen, nitrogen
  Hormones
  Enzymes
  Antibodies and antitoxins.

Plasma Proteins

Albumin is similar to the white of an egg. It is formed in the liver. Because it has a large molecular structure, it helps to retain water within the main bloodstream. It also assists in returning blood to the capillaries from the surrounding tissues.

Globulin is in two forms. One type is formed in the liver and assists in the transportation of lipids, hormones and trace elements. The second type, γ-globulin, is formed by the lymphocytes and is part of the immune system. It carries antibodies.

Prothrombin is also formed in the liver. This is one of the factors necessary for coagulation. Vitamin K is required to change it into thrombin.

Fibrinogen is also produced in the liver. Whenever coagulation of blood occurs, several things happen. Thrombin acts on fibrinogen, changing it into *fibrin*. This becomes fine filaments which form a mesh, trapping blood cells The fibrin then contracts and the serum binds everything together to form a clot.

Plasma is serum which contains fibrinogen. *Serum* is plasma without fibrinogen. Serum still contains the proteins, minerals and antibodies found in plasma.

Erythrocytes (Red Corpuscles)

These are the most numerous cells in the blood. There are $5–5\frac{1}{2}$ million per cubic millimetre of blood in the adult male, slightly less in the female. They may be described as biconcave, circular discs of approximately 7.5 thousandths of a millimetre. Because they do not have a nucleus the correct term for them is *corpuscle*, not cell.

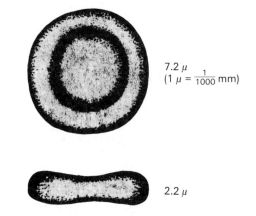

7.2μ
$(1 \mu = \frac{1}{1000}$ mm$)$

2.2μ

Erythrocytes (red blood corpuscles)

Erythrocytes contain the compound haemoglobin. This consists of a protein called globin combined with an iron-containing pigment called *haem* which gives the red colour to erythrocytes. When haemoglobin is combined with oxygen it makes *oxyhaemoglobin*. The colour is bright red, as in arterial blood. When there is a reduced amount of oxygen, as in the veins, the colour is a bluish purple.

Erythrocytes are formed in the red bone marrow. In young children, this is found in all cancellous bones.

By adulthood this has receded to the ends of the long bones, the sternum, ribs, skull and vertebrae. Vitamin B12 has been found to be an essential substance required for the development of mature erythrocytes. Without it, the erythrocytes do not form properly and a condition known as *pernicious anaemia* develops.

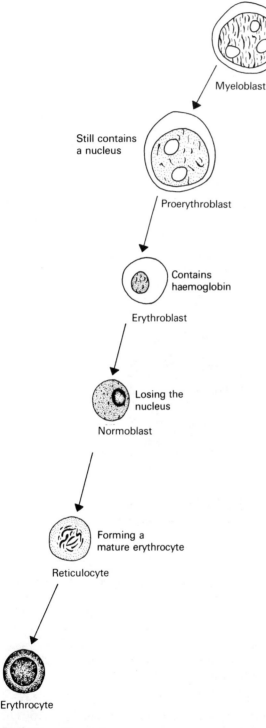

Erythrocyte formation

The lifespan of an erythrocyte is approximately 120 days. When they are broken down, the iron is stored for future re-use to produce haemoglobin.

Leucocytes (White Blood Cells)

These differ from erythrocytes in that they possess a nucleus, are colourless and less numerous. There are two categories of leucocytes: *granular* (polymorphonuclear) leucocytes and *non-granular* (mononuclear) *leucocytes*.

Granular (Polymorphonuclear) Leucocytes

These form 75 per cent of the white cells. They are irregular in shape and are capable of independent movement rather like an amoeba. The nucleus is irregular and the size can vary. There are small granules in the cytoplasm. The functions of the leucocytes are to defend the body against foreign micro-organisms and to act as scavengers by removing dead tissue. There are three types: neutrophils, eosinophils and basophils.

They all originate from the same myeloblasts as the erythrocytes. They undergo similar changes but keep their nuclei. They are named after the different dyes which stain the granules in laboratory tests.

Eosinophils respond to a red acid dye called *eosin*.
Basophils respond to a blue alkaline dye called *methylene blue*.
Neutrophils respond to both dyes and become purple in colour and have a neutral reaction.

Neutrophils
These form up to 70 per cent of the total number of leucocytes. They have a lifespan of about 30 hours. Their function is to lead the defence against invading micro-organisms. They are transported to an infected area through the walls of capillaries by a process known as *diapedesis*. Then they surround and ingest the organism in a process called *phagocytosis*. Within the cells are lysosomes which then digest and destroy the phagocytosed organisms.

Eosinophils
These form up to 6 per cent of the total number of leucocytes and are said to increase in number as a response to certain allergic conditions such as asthma and hayfever. They are thought to destroy antigen-antibody complexes. They are reduced in number when hydrocortisone levels are increased.

Basophils
These form only 2 per cent of the total number of leucocytes. They are sometimes called *mast cells*. It is thought that histamine and the anticoagulant *heparin* may be produced by them.

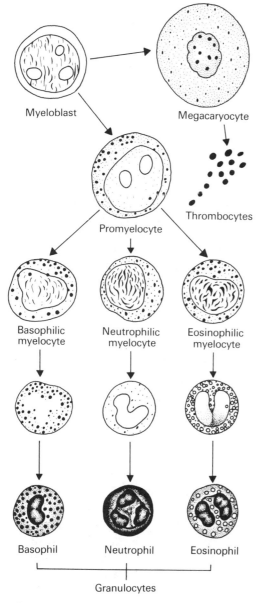

Development of granular leucocyte

Non-granular (Mononuclear) Leucocytes
These form 25 per cent of the white cells. There are two types: *monocytes* and *lymphocytes*.

Lymphocytes
These have a large round nucleus which fills most of the cell body. They are formed in the bone marrow and are stored in the lymph glands and spleen. Their lifespan may be from 2 to 200 days depending on their function. Lymphocytes may be classified as B-types or T-types.

B-type Lymphocytes travel freely around the body in both the blood and lymphatic systems. They appear to have the ability to search out foreign cells. They form specific antibodies which will only act against one particular antigen.

T-type Lymphocytes are stored in the thymus and are under the influence of hormones. They are transported to the lymph glands by the blood and lymph vessels. Their main function appears to be the rejection of foreign or transplanted tissue. They therefore form part of the immune system.

Monocytes
Monocytes are larger than lymphocytes but only form 2–8 per cent of the white cell count. They have a large nucleus and many lysosomes. They act as phagocytes on unwanted protein.

Platelets

These are small, disc-shaped bodies. They do not possess a nucleus but do contain granules within the protoplasm. Their function is to assist in blood clotting. When an injury occurs, *thromboplastin* is released by the damaged tissues. This substance converts *prothrombin* into *thrombin* which then acts to change *fibrinogen* into *fibrin*. This forms fibrous strands in which the platelets become enmeshed.

THE LYMPHATIC SYSTEM

This is a second circulatory system. It is closely associated with the blood system.

It consists of:

    lymph vessels
    lymph nodes
    lymph.

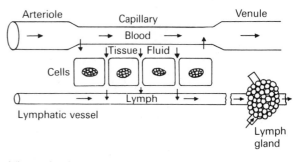

Tissue fluid exchange

Lymph Vessels

Just as the blood system has capillaries, so does the lymphatic system. These start as blind-ended channels in all the body tissues. They join larger lymph channels which ultimately converge into two large ducts called the *thoracic duct* and the *right lymphatic duct*.

The lymph capillaries are composed of a single layer of endothelial cells. The lymph channels consist of three layers. The inner lining consists of a single layer of endothelial cells. The middle layer is composed of muscular and elastic tissue while the outer layer consists of fibrous tissue which forms a protective covering.

Lymph is not pumped around the body like the blood. Instead, it relies on pressure from outside the lymph vessels to propel it along. Like the veins, the larger vessels have valves which prevent the lymph from flowing backwards.

The lymphatic duct collects all the lymph and returns it to the blood system. The lymph from the legs, the abdomen, the left side of the chest, the left arm and left side of the head is collected into a dilated sac which forms the *cisterna chyli*. This is about 40 cm (16 inches) long. It lies between the second lumbar vertebra and the root of the neck. It feeds into the venous system through the thoracic duct.

The right lymphatic duct is approximately 13 mm ($\frac{1}{2}$ inch) long and lies at the root of the neck. It collects lymph from the right arm, the right side of the chest and the right side of the head.

The ducts both discharge into the venous system at a point between the left and right internal jugular and the subclavian veins. These are guarded by semilunar valves which prevent blood from entering the lymphatic system.

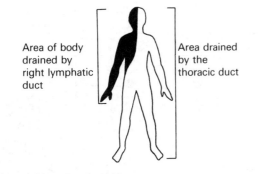

Area of lymphatic drainage

Lymph Nodes

Situated around the body are a number of lymph nodes. They vary in size from a pinhead to an almond. They may be oval, round or kidney-shaped. They usually occur in groups. Their numbers are reduced in old age. Some of the nodes are superficial but many lie deep in the body.

The body of the lymph node consists of a fine mesh of *reticulin* fibres called the *reticulum*. The lymphocytes and macrophages are held here in great numbers. Surrounding the node is a *capsule* composed mainly of collagen fibres. Several small lymph channels enter the node. They are called *afferent* vessels. Leaving the node is a single channel called an *efferent* vessel. It emerges from the central part of the node called the *medulla* through a small cavity called the *hilum*.

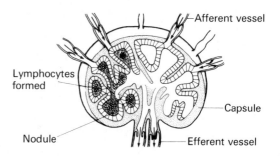

A lymph node

Lymph nodes act as filters to trap micro-organisms and damaged cells collected by the lymph. These are then broken down and destroyed by the lymphoid tissue. Lymphocytes (page 61) are stored in the nodes. They increase rapidly in number in times of both local and general infection.

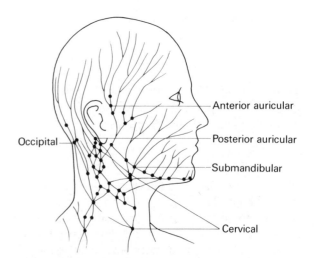

Lymph nodes and vessels of the head

Lymphatic tissue is found in other organs of the body. These include the tonsils and adenoids, the spleen, the appendix, Peyer's patches (in the wall of the small intestines) and the thymus. The thymus plays an important role in the development of lymphatic tissue as well as being the site for T-type lymphocyte activity.

Lymph

The composition of lymph is very similar to blood plasma. It also contains waste particles which are too large for the veins to carry, as well as material which could be damaging to the body. For example, when phagocytosis has occurred, the lymph will carry far more monocytes and neutrophils than usual.

DISORDERS OF THE BLOOD AND LYMPHATIC SYSTEMS

Aneurysm The wall of a blood vessel is stretched and becomes very thin.

Blood Poisoning (Septicaemia) May be local (when only a small area is infected) or general (when the whole body is affected). It is caused by micro-organisms and bacteria entering the blood system.

Broken Capillaries A rupturing of the walls of superficial capillaries.

Chilblains An inflamed condition of the skin caused by poor circulation to that area. It usually affects the hands and feet.

Epistaxis Bleeding from the nose.

Hypertension Above average blood pressure.

Hypotension Below average blood pressure.

Thrombus A clot of blood found within the blood system.

Lymphadenitis An inflammation of lymph glands.

Lymphangitis An inflammation of the lymph vessels.

Lymphoedema An accumulation of lymph causing swelling in an organ; due to the obstruction of the lymph vessels draining it.

Hodgkin's Disease (Lymphadenoma) A condition where all the lymph glands gradually enlarge. Anaemia is prevalent and the patient becomes gradually weaker.

Anaemia A condition of the blood, due to quantitative and qualitative changes in the erythrocytes. There are a number of forms this condition may take:

Simple Anaemia A deficiency of erythrocytes. It may be caused by loss of blood, defective formation of erythrocytes, an inadequate intake of iron or the body's inability to absorb iron.

Pernicious Anaemia Caused by lack of an essential anti-pernicious factor normally produced in the body, necessary for forming normoblasts in the marrow.

Aplastic Anaemia This occurs when the bone marrow ceases to produce erythrocytes.

Haemolytic Anaemia This is caused by excessive destruction of erythrocytes, usually by the action of poisonous substances.

Sickle-Cell Anaemia This is due to the presence of an abnormal form of haemoglobin, which makes erythrocytes sickle-shaped. It is usually found only in people native to the equatorial tropics.

Chapter 8

The Endocrine System

This system is sometimes referred to as the *ductless gland system*. It consists of a number of glands in different areas on the body. They do not have ducts but pour their secretions directly into the bloodstream. These secretions are known as *hormones*.

Once in the bloodstream, a hormone travels until it reaches the target cells of some distant organ. Some hormones like *adrenalin* may have an instant effect. Others are associated with growth and take many years to produce any effect. Some glands may produce more than one hormone.

The endocrine system consists of:
   the pituitary gland
   the pineal gland
   the thyroid gland
   four parathyroid glands
   two adrenal (suprarenal) glands
   the islets of Langerhans in the pancreas
   two ovaries (in the female) or two testes (in the male).

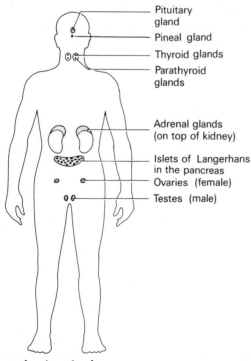

Pituitary gland
Pineal gland
Thyroid glands
Parathyroid glands
Adrenal glands (on top of kidney)
Islets of Langerhans in the pancreas
Ovaries (female)
Testes (male)

The endocrine glands

THE PITUITARY GLAND (HYPOPHYSIS)

This gland is situated in the hypophyseal fossa at the base of the brain. It is joined to the hypothalamus area of the brain by a stalk, placed just behind the optic chiasma. It is oval in shape, approximately 15 mm ($\frac{5}{8}$ inch) long and 5 mm ($\frac{1}{4}$ inch) across. It is greyish-red in colour. The pituitary gland is formed from two lobes; the *anterior* and the *posterior* lobes. Although under the control of the hypothalamus, the lobes have quite different functions.

The Anterior Lobe (Adenohypophysis)

The hypothalamus produces releasing factors that affect certain hormones. This lobe produces six hormones:

   thyroid-stimulating hormone (TSH)
   corticotrophin (adrenocorticotrophic) hormone (ACTH)
   growth hormone (GH)
   follicle-stimulating hormone (FSH)
   luteinizing hormone (LH)
   prolactin (PRL).

Thyroid-stimulating Hormone (TSH)

This hormone stimulates the *thyroid gland* into activity. It also controls the growth of the thyroid gland. The release of TSH by the pituitary gland is stimulated by the hypothalamus releasing its thyrotrophin-releasing hormone (TRH).

Corticotrophin (Adrenocorticotrophic) Hormone (ACTH)

This hormone stimulates the cortex of the *adrenal gland* into producing a *steroid* called *cortisol*. This steroid can provide a negative feedback to the hypothalamus when the hormonal level drops, and may also stimulate the production of other steroids. ACTH also controls the pigmentation of melanocytes which give the skin its natural colour.

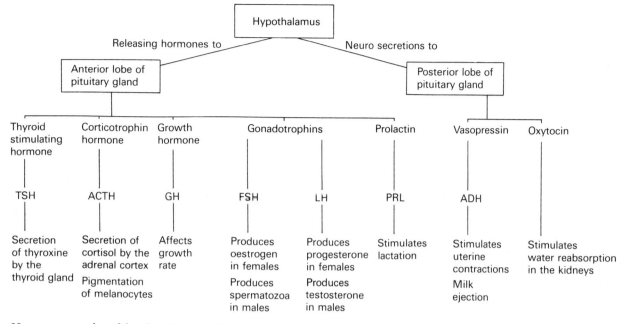

Hormones produced by the pituitary gland

Growth Hormone (GH)

This hormone is also known as *somatotrophin*. It influences the liver into producing proteins called *somatomedins*. These have the effect of increasing the growth rate. The hypothalamus can also release somatostatin, which inhibits growth rate.

The following two hormones are known as *gonadotrophins*.

Follicle-stimulating Hormone (FSH)

In the female, FSH causes the ovarian follicles to ripen and so produce *oestrogen*. In the male, FSH initiates the production of *spermatozoa*.

The Luteinizing Hormone (LH)

This causes the formation of the corpus luteum which produces *progesterone* in the female. In the male, the interstitial cells in the testes are stimulated into producing *testosterone*.

Prolactin (PRL)

This hormone promotes lactation in the nursing mother. The production of prolactin is stimulated by the sucking of a baby. When the sucking ceases, lactation also ceases.

The Posterior Pituitary Lobe (Neurohypophysis)

This part of the pituitary gland responds to neural stimulation from the hypothalamus. Two hormones are produced in this lobe. They are:

    vasopressin
    oxytocin.

Vasopressin (Antidiuretic Hormone: ADH)

This hormone's main function is to stimulate the kidneys into concentrating urine and thereby reducing its volume. The excess fluid is reabsorbed into the bloodstream. Another function of ADH is to maintain the osmotic pressure of plasma. When there is a rise in plasma osmolality or a low plasma volume (caused by the kidneys retaining extra fluid in their tubules), extra ADH is released. The kidneys then release their fluid into the bloodstream. Conversely, as osmotic pressure rises in the blood vessels, the amount of ADH secretion is reduced and more urine is produced.

A further function is to cause the involuntary muscles of the blood vessels, urinary bladder and intestines to contract. This can raise the blood pressure, especially in times of stress, pain, or when certain drugs or alcohol are present. A deficiency of ADH can cause diabetes insipidus.

Oxytocin

This hormone has two functions. It stimulates the uterine muscles to contract during childbirth. It also acts to contract the *myo-epithelial cells* in the breasts, squeezing milk into the lactiferous ducts behind the nipples.

THE PINEAL GLAND

This gland lies in the mid-line of the brain, just behind the third ventricle. It is about the size of a pea and is reddish-grey in colour.

Its functions are not fully understood. It is believed to play an inhibiting or regulating role in the activities of the pituitary gland and possibly the gonads until puberty. It is also thought to play a role in coordinating the circadian rhythms.

THE THYROID GLAND

This gland lies at the lower part of the throat. It consists of two lobes which lie on either side of the trachea. The two lobes are joined by an isthmus just below the cricoid cartilage. The lobes are conical in shape being approximately 3 cm ($\frac{1}{4}$ inches) wide and 5 cm (2 inches) long. The whole gland is covered by a fibrous capsule and is brownish-red in colour. It is supplied by numerous blood vessels.

The thyroid gland contains two types of cell: the *follicular* cells and the *parafollicular* (clear) cells.

Follicular Cells

These produce the hormones called:
  iodothyronine (T_3)
  thyroxine (T_4).

Iodothyronine and Thyroxine

The follicular cells are able to change their shape, which depends on whether they are being stimulated by the thyroid-stimulating hormone (TSH) produced by the pituitary gland. Between the cells are spaces called *alveoli*. These collect a thick, sticky substance called *thyroglobulin*. It is converted by the follicular cells into *iodothryonine*. This regulates the basal metabolic rate by controlling the utilisation of oxygen. It also influences growth, especially of nerve fibres.

This hormone, together with the less active *thyroxine*, takes up and stores iodine from the plentiful supply in the blood. This action produces a feedback to the hypothalamus. This in turn triggers the anterior lobe of the pituitary into producing or inhibiting the release of thyrotrophin-releasing hormone (TRH). Other functions of iodothyronine and thyroxine include: stimulation of absorption of carbohydrates from the small intestines, maintenance of healthy hair and skin, and heat production during the release of energy by the cells.

If there is a deficiency of iodine in the diet or hypersecretion of these hormones, the thyroid gland may enlarge to form a swelling known as a goitre. A condition called *thyrotoxicosis* may develop. Its symptoms include weight loss, nervousness, rapid pulse, increased sweating and the characteristic protrusion of the eyeballs.

Hyposecretion of thyroid hormones can lead to *cretinism* in infants, or *myxoedema* in adults. This lowers metabolism, causes speech or movement to be slow, dries the skin and lowers temperature. These people can often appear to be mentally slower.

Parafollicular (Clear) Cells

These produce the hormone called *calcitonin*.

Calcitonin

This hormone controls the calcium level in the blood. Its function is to reduce the level of calcium in the blood by preventing its reabsorption from bone.

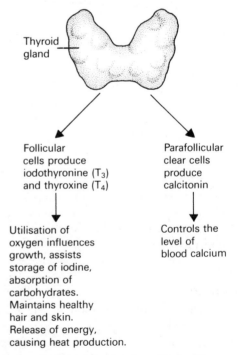

Hormones produced by the thyroid gland

THE PARATHYROID GLANDS

There are four small, ovoid glands of approximately 6 mm ($\frac{1}{4}$ inch) long. They usually lie in pairs behind the thyroid gland. They are a brownish-yellow in colour. The function of these glands is to secrete a hormone called *parathormone*.

Parathormone

The function of parathormone is to both control and raise the level of calcium in the blood. It acts in the opposite manner to calcitonin (produced by the thyroid gland).

Calcium is needed by the body, in particular for the cardiac and striated muscles. If the level of the calcium in the blood serum is too low, these muscles can go into spasm in a condition called *tetany*. To counteract this, the body may increase production of parathormone. If this occurs too often it can raise the calcium level to a critical height, so that renal calculi (kidney stones) and bone disease may occur.

THE ADRENAL (SUPRARENAL) GLANDS

These two glands lie just above each of the two kidneys. They are approximately 5 cm (2 inches) long and 3 cm ($1\frac{1}{2}$ inches) wide. They are roughly the shape of a pyramid and are yellowish in colour. They have a rich blood supply with arterial blood being drawn from the large abdominal aorta and the renal arteries. The right gland drains into the inferior vena cava and the left gland drains into the left renal vein.

Each adrenal gland is divided into two parts: *the cortex* (outer part) and *the medulla* (inner part).

The Adrenal Cortex

This part completely surrounds the medulla. It produces three types of hormones called *steroids*. This is because of their waxy appearance. The three types are classified as:

> glucocorticoids
> mineralocorticoids
> sex hormones.

Glucocorticoids

The three main steroids (hormones) in this group are: *cortisol* (hydrocortisone), *corticosterone* and *11-deoxycortisol*.

The adrenal cortex is stimulated into producing these three steroids by the action of ACTH (produced in the anterior lobe of the pituitary gland). The main functions of glucocorticoids are:

1 to regulate carbohydrate metabolism
2 to maintain the output of glucose by the liver
3 to increase the output of glucose in times of stress
4 to be responsible for changing glycogen into glucose
5 to mobilise lipids (fat) from the tissues
6 to increase the breakdown (catabolism) of proteins
7 to suppress the growth hormone (GH) from the anterior lobe of the pituitary
8 to reduce the number of eosinophils and lymphocytes in the blood
9 to increase the number of neutrophils in the blood
10 to suppress the immune system
11 to reduce inflammation
12 to reduce the effect of vitamin D so that absorption of calcium in the small intestines is decreased.

Synthetically-prepared cortisone, which is converted by the body into hydrocortisone, is often administered to suppress inflammation. However, the side-effects may result in an imbalance of salt and water in the body fluids.

Mineralocorticoids

The main mineralocorticoid is called *aldosterone*.

Aldosterone regulates the amount of sodium and potassium in the body. This maintains the ion levels which balance the fluids and electrolytes.

Aldosterone stimulates the renal tubules into reabsorbing sodium. This increases the amount of potassium present. Any excess of potassium is excreted.

The Sex Hormones

Small quantities of both the male hormones, *androgens*, and the female hormones, *oestrogens*, are produced in the cortex. They are produced in greater amounts until puberty when the testes and ovaries mature. They are controlled by ACTH. The adrenal cortex is the main source of androgens in the female. Both hormones influence the development of secondary sex characteristics.

The Adrenal Medulla

The medulla is surrounded by the adrenal cortex. It secretes two hormones called *adrenalin* and *noradrenalin*. The secretion of these is controlled by the sympathetic nervous system. Noradrenalin is a nerve chemical transmitter, transmitting nerve impulses ('messages') along a nerve. They are known as the hormones of 'flight or fright' because in these situations the hormones are secreted in large quantitites. They are responsible for emotional stimulations, bringing heightened sensitivity and awareness during periods of excitement.

The main effects of adrenalin and noradrenalin are:

1 relaxation of the bronchi muscles – increasing the intake of oxygen
2 constriction of the arterioles in the body – raising the blood pressure, and increasing both the heart rate and the force of the heartbeat
3 stimulation of the liver – converting glycogen into glucose (needed by the muscles)
4 reduction of salivary secretions – causing the mouth to become dry, and slowing peristalsis in the intestines
5 increase of activity in the sweat glands and contraction of arrector pili muscles – causing 'goose pimples'.

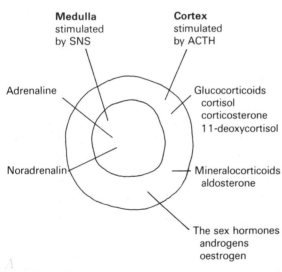

Secretions of the adrenal gland

THE ISLETS OF LANGERHANS

The islets of Langerhans are made up of clusters of cells. They are found throughout the pancreas. There are three cell types: *alpha* cells, *beta* cells and *delta* cells.

Alpha Cells

These cells secrete a hormone called *glucagon*. It acts on glycogen in the liver converting this into glucose, which is then released into the blood system.

The normal level of glucose in the blood is between 3.4 and 5.5 mmol per litre. When the glucose level falls, more glucagon is released.

Beta Cells

The hormone released by these cells is called *insulin*. This acts in the opposite manner to glucagon, converting glucose to glycogen: reducing the glucose level in the blood. Insulin acts on the cell walls so that glucose may enter the cells, where it is catabolised as energy and heat, and converted into glycogen; which may be stored in the muscles or liver. Insulin also inhibits the breaking down of fats and promotes the synthesis of proteins.

A deficiency of insulin can lead to a condition called *diabetes mellitus*. This results in a high blood glucose level, and may also result in a poor metabolism of fat.

Delta Cells

These cells secrete a hormone called *somatostatin*, which is also secreted by the hypothalamus. It is able to inhibit the secretion of a number of other hormones, one of which is the growth hormone (secreted by the pituitary). Somatostatin is therefore known as the *growth hormone release inhibiting hormone (GHRIH)*.

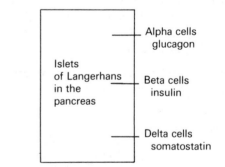

Secretions from the islets of Langerhans

THE OVARIES

These two glands lie on the lateral wall of the pelvis. They are part of the female reproductive system. The ovaries have a cycle of activity which lasts approximately 28 days. They produce three hormones: *oestrogen*, *progesterone* and *androgens*.

Oestrogen

This hormone is needed for the development of secondary sexual characteristics at puberty. It is required later for the development of the female reproductive organs and the stimulation of the mammary glands.

Progesterone

This hormone can only have an effect on tissues previously stimulated by oestrogen.

The main effect is to change the endometrium (uterus lining) prior to pregnancy. A secondary effect is the enlargement of the alveolar cells of the breast prior to producing milk.

Androgens

This hormone is secreted in small amounts and is utilised in the body for the development of secondary sexual characteristics. A surfeit of androgens in a female can produce an excess of hair on the face and body and a typically masculine body shape.

THE TESTES

These two glands form part of the male reproductive system. They lie within the *scrotal sac*. The main hormone produced by them is called *testosterone*. Two other, lesser, hormones are also produced. The male hormones are known collectively as *androgens*.

Until puberty, very little testosterone is secreted. At the time of puberty, the anterior lobe of the pituitary starts to secrete the *luteinizing hormone* (LH). This stimulates the interstitial cells into producing testosterone.

Testosterone produces marked changes in the body. They include:

1 hair starting to grow on the face, chest, abdomen and pubis
2 an enlargement of the larynx; which causes the voice to 'break' and become deeper
3 maturation of the sex organs and the production of spermatozoa
4 stimulation of protein synthesis so that bones become larger and muscles are increased in size and strength.

Chapter 9

Accessory Organs: the Hands, Feet, Nails, Hair and Breasts

THE HANDS

Bones of the Lower Arm and Hand

The bones of the lower arm are the *radius* and *ulna*. The radius is the larger of the two bones. It lies on the inner aspect of the arm on the same side as the thumb.

The radius and ulna articulate with the eight bones of the wrist. These are known collectively as *carpals*. They are arranged in two rows.

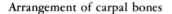

Thumb	Fingers		Little finger
Trapezium	Trapezoid	Capitate	Hamate
Scaphoid	Lunate	Triquetral	Pisiform
Radius		Ulna	

Arrangement of carpal bones

The carpals are eight small, irregular, interlocking bones. They are held in position by ligaments. The movement between any two bones is small but there is great flexibility when they are all moved together.

The second or *distal* row of carpals articulate with the five *metacarpals* that form the hand. Although small, they are classified as *long bones*. They each have a *shaft*, a *base* and a *head*. There is greater mobility between the *trapezium* and the first metacarpal (the thumb) than any other of the joints. The thumb lies anterior to the other metacarpals and is able to rotate, allowing it to touch all the other fingers.

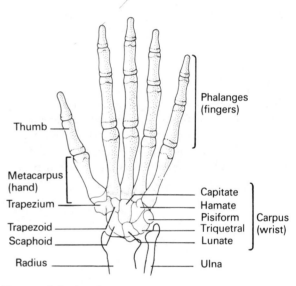

Bones of the hand

The metacarpals articulate with the *phalanges* that form the fingers and thumb. The thumb has only two phalanges while the fingers have three: a *proximal*, a *middle* and a *distal* phalanx (singular). These are also classified as long bones.

The Muscles of the Lower Arm and Hand

The muscles that move the wrist and hand joints have their points of origin in the upper arm. The distal ends form strong ligaments so that the points of insertion are in the fingertips. The ligaments are held close to the wrist by a strong capsular ligament formed by the *thenar* and *hypothenar* muscles which surround the wrist.

The main muscles moving the hand and wrist are:
flexor carpi radialis – flexes the wrist joint
extensor carpi radialis – extends the wrist
flexor carpi ulnaris – flexes the wrist
extensor carpi ulnaris – extends the wrist.

These four muscles also cause the movements of abduction (towards the body) and adduction (away from the body). Other muscles include:

flexor digitorum – flexes the fingers
extensor digitorum – extends the fingers.

ANTERIOR ASPECT

POSTERIOR ASPECT

Muscles of the lower arm and hand

The Vascular System of the Hand

Arteries

One of the main arteries of the upper arm is the *brachial* artery. It divides at the elbow into the *radial* and *ulnar* arteries. These pass in front of the wrist and interlink to form the deep and superficial *palmar arches*. Leaving these are the *digital* arteries to each finger where they become arterial capillaries.

Veins

The venous capillaries lead into many superficial veins. These are most numerous at the back of the hands. They pass into the *cephalic* and the *median* veins. At the elbow the median vein goes into the *basilic* vein and then into the *axillary* vein. The

cephalic vein is joined by the *accessory cephalic* vein to form the *brachial* vein. These join other veins and then form the *subclavian* vein.

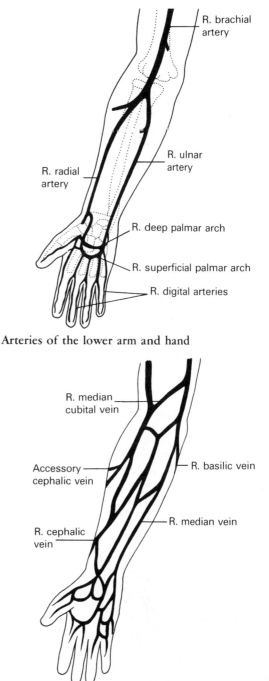

Arteries of the lower arm and hand

Veins of the lower arm and hand

Lymph Vessels

The hand and lower arm contain a network of lymph vessels. These pass through the *supratrochlear* nodes situated at the front of the elbow. The next major group of nodes that they pass through are the *axillary* nodes.

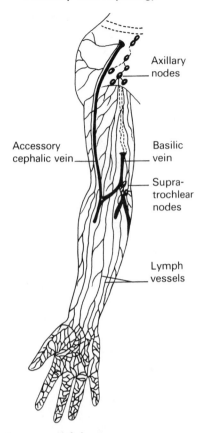

Lymphatic system of the arm

Nerves of the Lower Arm and Hand

There are three main nerves which supply the lower arm and the hand. They are: the *radial*, the *ulnar* and the *median* nerves. The ulnar nerve lies superficially on the outer edge of the humerus at the elbow. This has caused the area to become known as the 'funny bone'.

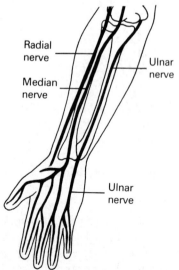

Nerves of the lower arm and hand

THE FEET

Bones of the Lower Leg and Foot

The bones of the lower leg are the *tibia* and the *fibula*. The tibia is the larger of the two bones. It lies medially or inside the fibula and forms the shin bone.

The ankle joint is formed by the tibia articulating over the *talus* and the fibula. The posterior part of the foot is made up of seven small, irregular bones called *tarsal* bones. These are held in place by a number of tendons and ligaments. The largest tarsal bone is the *calcaneus*. This forms the heel bone.

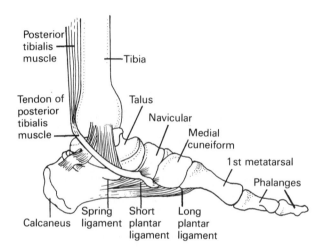

Ligaments and tendons supporting the arch of the foot

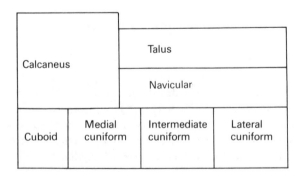

Tarsal bones

Articulating with the tarsal bones are five *metatarsal* bones. These articulate with fourteen *phalanges* which form the toes.

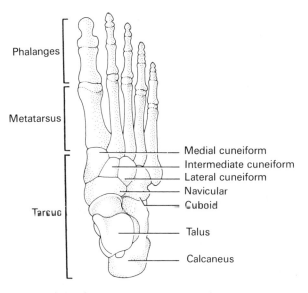

Phalanges

Metatarsus

Tarsus

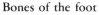

Medial cuneiform
Intermediate cuneiform
Lateral cuneiform
Navicular
Cuboid
Talus
Calcaneus

Bones of the foot

The Vascular System of the Lower Leg and Foot

Arteries

The main arteries of the lower leg are the anterior and posterior *tibial* arteries, and the *peroneal* artery. The anterior tibial artery feeds into the *dorsalis pedis* artery and thence into the *digital* arteries of the toes. The posterior tibial and the peroneal arteries supply the plantar arch on the sole of the foot.

Muscles of the Lower Leg and Foot

The main muscles of the lower leg are the *gastrocnemius*, the *soleus*, the *anterior tibialis* and the *peroneus longus*. They allow the ankle to be moved in all directions. The flexor and extensor *digitorum longus* cause the toes to move. The tendons passing over the front of the ankle are held in place by two strong bands of tendinous tissue called the *anterior talofibular ligament*. The broad tendon of the gastrocnemius is inserted into the calcaneus. It is known as the *achilles tendon*.

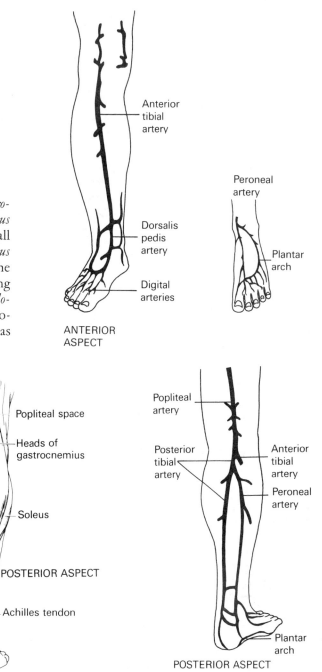

Anterior tibial artery

Dorsalis pedis artery

Digital arteries

ANTERIOR ASPECT

Peroneal artery

Plantar arch

Patella bone

Tendon of rectus femoris

Sartorius tendon

Gastrocnemius

Tibialis anterior
Peroneous longus

Extensor digitorum longus

Soleus

ANTERIOR ASPECT

Medial malleolus bone

Calcaneum bone

Muscles of the lower leg and foot

Popliteal space

Heads of gastrocnemius

Soleus

POSTERIOR ASPECT

Achilles tendon

Popliteal artery

Posterior tibial artery

Anterior tibial artery

Peroneal artery

Plantar arch

POSTERIOR ASPECT

Arteries of the lower leg and foot

Veins

There are two main superficial veins in the lower leg. Blood is collected from capillaries under the foot and passes into the *short saphenous* vein. Behind the knee this passes into the *popliteal* vein. Blood from the front of the foot and leg passes upwards through the *long saphenous* vein to the *femoral* vein.

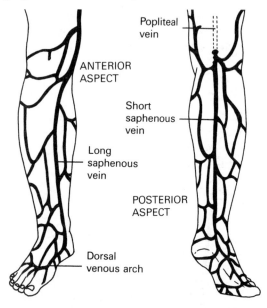

Veins of the lower leg and foot

Lymph Vessels

Lymph is collected in a series of canals and transported to the *popliteal* node at the back of the knee before continuing up to the *inguinal* nodes.

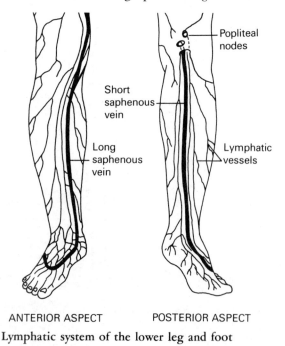

Lymphatic system of the lower leg and foot

Nerves of the Lower Leg and Foot

The main nerve at the front of the leg is the *femoral* nerve. This passes into the *saphenous* nerve. In the posterior aspect, the *sciatic* nerve travels right down the leg. It branches to form the *common peroneal*, *tibial* and *sural* nerves. These also supply the anterior aspect of the lower leg and foot.

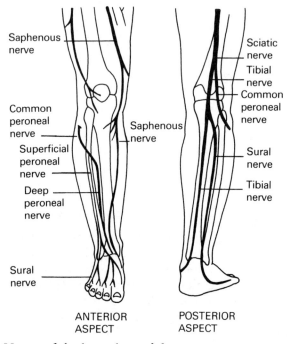

Nerves of the lower leg and foot

THE NAILS

At the end of the fingers and toes are pads of specialised horny cells which form the nails. Other animals and birds have similar structures, such as hooves or claws. Nails protect the ends of the fingers and form a stiff backing to the soft, sensitive pulp of the fingertips. The stubby finger ends seen in people who continually bite their nails results from the loss of this stiffening.

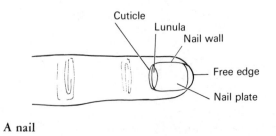

A nail

The Nail Plate

This is dead, horny tissue. It is formed from hard, dry *keratinous* cells that have little moisture or fat. Nails have a high sulphur content, tending to split when the sulphur level is reduced. In order to keep the nails strong and healthy, the diet should contain sufficient amounts of sulphur, amino acids, phosphates and calcium. These are found in meat, cheese, milk and eggs. A pink colour showing through the nail is usually an indication of good health. A blue colour often indicates poor circulation.

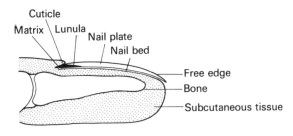

Cross-section of a nail

The Matrix

This is the most important part of the nail. It is the area where new cells are produced to form the nail plate. Numerous blood vessels and nerve endings supply it. Severe damage to the matrix may stop the growth of the new nail or make it grow in a distorted manner.

The Lunula

This is the whitish, opaque area at the base of the nail. It forms the halfmoon. The pale appearance is due to the fact that it does not adhere so closely to the underlying tissue. It might be called the 'bridge' between the living matrix and the closely packed layer of cells which comprise the nail plate.

The Cuticle

This is a fold of skin lying over the matrix area. The edge of it is formed from dry, keratinous cells. Unless cared for, it will adhere to the nail and grow out with it. This can result in a tear. A similar fold of skin lies along the sides of the nail. Together they are known as the *nail wall*.

The Free Edge

This is the part of the nail plate that has grown longer than the nail bed.

The Nail Bed

This is the part of the finger that lies under the nail plate. It contains numerous fine blood capillaries.

The appearance of the nails changes with age and the state of health. In young adults they are usually smooth and free of ridges and grooves. They should be neither brittle nor too soft. In old age they are likely to become more brittle and rather opaque. They often become thickened and rough, and may be ridged. The growth rate of a nail varies. The average is approximately 3 mm ($\frac{1}{8}$ inch) per month. It takes four to six months to produce a completely new nail. The toenails take longer. Nails grow faster in summer and in young people.

HAIR

Hairs are dead, keratinised structures. They are formed in the dermis of the skin in a tube-like structure called a *follicle*.

A follicle starts as an indentation of the surface of the epidermis and is continuous with it. It has two layers. The outer is made of fibrous tissue and is highly vascular, with numerous nerves. The inner layer is itself formed by two layers of cells called the outer and inner *root sheath*. The outer root sheath is similar in structure to the stratum spinosum (see page 21) and forms the wall of the follicle. At the base of the follicle the cells become continuous with those of the hair root.

The inner root sheath consists of three layers of cells, some having a flattened nucleus, others having none at all. When the hair grows longer and deeper, the follicle elongates to accommodate it.

The part of the hair that grows above the surface of the epidermis is called the *hair shaft*.

The part of the hair that grows within the follicle is called the *hair root*. The enlarged end is called the

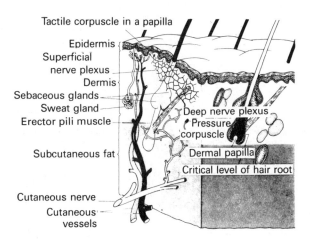

Section of a hair in a follicle

bulb. The growth cells of the hair are found here. It is surrounded by a structure of loose connective tissue called the *dermal papilla*. It receives nourishment directly from the dermal capillaries and in turn nourishes the hair bulb.

Emptying into most hair follicles is a sebaceous gland which secretes sebum.

Hairs do not grow out straight from the skin; they grow at an angle. There is an involuntary muscle attached to the underside of the hair follicle, lying in the same direction as the hair grows. When cold or fear is felt, this muscle pulls the hair follicle so that the hair stands on end. It also produces 'goose pimples'. The name of the muscle is *erector pili* (or *arrectores pilorum* in the plural).

Hair has been given different names on the various parts of the body:
  capilli – hairs on the head
  supercilia – eyebrows
  cilia – eyelashes
  barba – facial hair
  hirci – axillary hair
  pubes – hairs on the pubis.

Types of Hair

There are two main kinds of hair: vellus and terminal hair. A foetus may also have lanugo hairs, which are discarded just after birth.

Vellus Hairs

These are soft, downy hairs found all over the body except on the palms of the hands and soles of the feet. They grow from a very shallow follicle, often from the edge of a sebaceous gland. They receive their nourishment from this gland rather than from the dermal papilla and therefore have a very elementary bulb. They are not normally pigmented, remaining blonde in colour. Vellus hairs normally have a very slow rate of growth. They do not normally change into terminal hair unless subjected to external stimuli. Vellus hairs do not contain a medulla.

Terminal Hairs

The hairs found on the scalp, eyebrows, axilla and pubis differ from the vellus hairs and are called terminal hairs. They are much coarser and grow from a much deeper level in the dermis than vellus hair. They have well-developed bulbs and dermal papillae which are lacking in vellus hairs.

Terminal hair consists of three concentric layers of cells:

1 The *medulla* is the inner core. It is composed of keratinised cells interspersed with air spaces and some cells containing air. The air cells give terminal hair lightness and flexibility.

2 The *cortex* surrounds the medulla. This layer consists of elongated cells, held together, and containing granules of the pigment *melanin*. This gives the hair colour. The melanin may not reach to the end of the hair, making it appear pale. White or pale hairs with no melanin granules have air cells instead.

3 The *cuticle* is the outer layer. It consists of a single layer of overlapping flat cells. They do not contain any pigment.

The life of a hair is approximately four months. Eyelashes are replaced more frequently; while it takes about four years for a capilli hair to grow. The speed at which hair grows varies from about 1.5 mm ($\frac{1}{16}$ inch) per week for fine hair to 2.2 mm ($\frac{3}{32}$ inch) per week for coarse hair. Straight hairs are either round or oval in shape and are stronger than curly hairs which are flat.

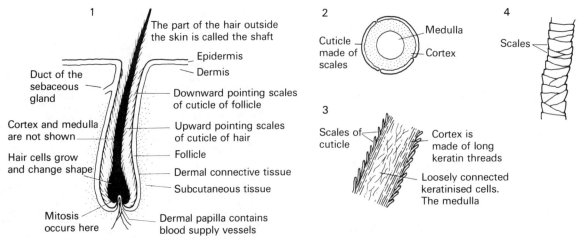

1

The part of the hair outside the skin is called the shaft

Duct of the sebaceous gland

Cortex and medulla are not shown

Hair cells grow and change shape

Mitosis occurs here

Epidermis

Dermis

Downward pointing scales of cuticle of follicle

Upward pointing scales of cuticle of hair

Follicle

Dermal connective tissue

Subcutaneous tissue

Dermal papilla contains blood supply vessels

2

Cuticle made of scales

Medulla

Cortex

3

Scales of cuticle

Cortex is made of long keratin threads

Loosely connected keratinised cells. The medulla

4

Scales

Cross-section of a hair

Hair Growth

There are three main phases of hair growth. The follicle is said to be either in:

the *anagen* stage
the *catagen* stage or
the *telogen* stage.

Anagen Stage

This is the first stage: it is a period of growth. As the hair grows upwards from the bulb, the follicle grows deeper into the dermis.

Catagen Stage

This is the second stage, covering a very short period of time. The hair bulb becomes detached from the dermal papillae, but still receives its nourishment from the walls of the follicle. At this time the hair is known as a *club* hair. The follicle left below the bulb often collapses and then shrinks. The club hair continues to rise up to the level of the sebaceous gland. It then becomes completely detached and falls out.

Telogen Stage

This is the stage when the follicle is resting. It is when the new hair cells are waiting to be germinated from the cells of the outer root sheath and the dermal papillae. At times, late in the catagen stage when the club hair falls out, there may be a new hair already germinating. This means that the follicle returns to the anagen stage without having a telogen rest stage. Occasionally there may even be a new hair growing behind the club hair.

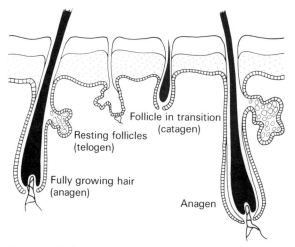

Stages of hair growth

Hair may be categorised as having either a normal or abnormal pattern. There are three main causes of hair growth: *congenital*, *topical* and *systemic*.

Congenital Growth

The congenital cause takes into account the hereditary factor as well as ethnic origins.

Protection

Hair is thought to have evolved to protect the human body. Hairs on the head serve to protect against knocks, to keep the rain and snow off and so retain heat. They can also prevent heatstroke by protecting the head from the sun's rays.

Eyebrows and eyelashes help to protect the eyes from bright sunlight and to stop dust from irritating the eyes. The hairs inside the nostrils help to filter dust out of the air and so protect the lungs. Hair at the axilla and pubis is there to protect against friction.

Males start to develop hair on their faces at puberty. They may also develop hairs inside their ears in their middle years.

All this is considered to be normal hair growth.

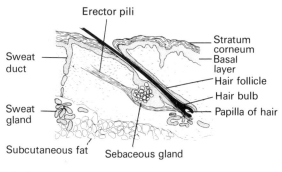

A hair

Genetics and Hair

Hair structure, colour and pattern are part of the personal genetic structure inherited from parents and forbears. This will determine colour, amount, and whether the hair is straight or curly, fine or coarse. All the males in some families may start to go bald early, while the women in other families may all develop superfluous hair on their faces. One family may produce very little body hair. Another family may produce an abundance of hair.

The distribution of hair varies between different ethnic groups. People of Anglo-Saxon, Nordic or Teutonic origin generally have less hair than Asians or people of mediterranean or semitic extraction. Generally Afro-Caribbean people have less hair than those of European origin, while the Oriental group, including Mongolians and American Indians, have least hair of all. What one group of people considers to be a normal or attractive amount of hair another group would consider quite unacceptable. In some countries, a woman with hair on her upper lip may be considered as normal. It would be very quickly removed in people of another culture.

'Beauty lies in the eye of the beholder.'

Very occasionally an abnormal amount of hair may be produced by an unfortunate genetic structure. A heavy growth may cover the entire body, except the palms of the hands and the soles of the feet. It may appear on the newborn infant or develop later in life.

The term *superfluous hair* simply means an excess or socially unacceptable amount of hair *for that person*. It may actually be a normal amount for the age and sex of that person.

Hypertrichosis is an abnormal amount of hair growing in areas that normally produce hair.

Hirsutism is an excessive growth of hair found on a part of the body not normally covered by hair.

Topical Growth

Topical causes of hair growth may be considered abnormal. They are normally localised. Hairs receive their nourishment through the dermal papillae or the wall of the follicles. Anything that causes a local irritation is likely to cause an increase in the blood supply to the skin and so bring increased nourishment to the hair follicles. A good example of this is when a limb is encased in plaster of Paris. The plaster has a rough feeling against the skin. There may be loose particles trapped under it. All this sets up an irritation. When the plaster is removed it is seen that extra hair has grown to protect the skin against this irritation. This topical growth will not normally be permanent.

Other causes of irritation are exposure to excessive, prolonged ultraviolet, and also rough winds. Agricultural workers who work outside in all weathers often show signs of additional hair growth. People who indulge in outdoor sporting activities often develop an acceleration of vellus growth, particularly on the nose, which often suffers from the effects of sunburn.

Moles and birthmarks have a naturally raised blood supply so that it is not unusual to find a crop of hairs growing from them. It is said that because of this accelerated cellular growth they may occasionally be carcinogenic. For this reason the hair should not be removed except under medical supervision.

Systemic Growth

The third cause of hair growth is of systemic origin. That is, the body itself stimulates its own hair growth as a result of over-stimulation of the endocrine system. The endocrine glands secrete hormones directly into the bloodstream (see Chapter 8).

If there is an over-production of androgens, superfluous hair or even hypertrichosis may result, particularly in the female. If there is an under-production of androgens, baldness may result, especially in the male.

THE BREASTS

The breasts or mammary glands are accessory glands of the female reproductive system. In children and in males they are in a very rudimentary state. The female breasts begin to develop at puberty when the hormones oestrogen and progesterone are produced.

The breast tissue consists of approximately twenty *lobes* separated by fibrous tissue. Each lobe is formed from a number of *lobules*. These lobules are separated by a fine network of connective tissue, where fat cells are deposited. The number of fat cells determines the size of the breasts. The shape varies considerably among women. The breasts lie over the pectoral muscles, and do not have much muscular support.

Within the lobules are clusters of secretory cells called *alveoli*. They open into small *ducts*. These in turn unite to form one larger duct called the *lactiferous* duct. This widens to form *lactiferous sinuses* just behind the nipple, which open on to the surface of the nipple.

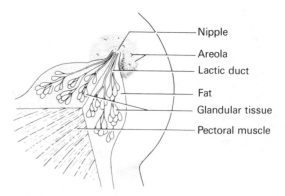

Nipple
Areola
Lactic duct
Fat
Glandular tissue
Pectoral muscle

Section through the breast

The breasts do not fully develop until pregnancy occurs. The mammary glands are only fully active during pregnancy and lactation.

The *nipple* is composed of erectile tissue covered by smooth epithelial tissue. It is surrounded by a pigmented area called the *areola*. This is usually pink or pale brown in colour but darkens during the first pregnancy.

The breasts have a good arterial and venous blood supply. There are also numerous lymph vessels which drain into the axillary lymph nodes.

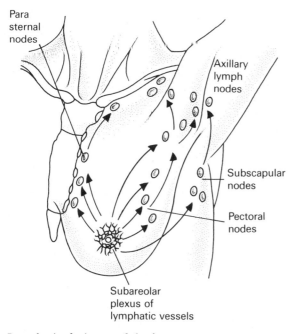

Lymphatic drainage of the breast

The breasts are supplied by the fourth, fifth and sixth thoracic nerves. There are numerous nerve endings particularly around the nipples, which especially respond to the sucking of a baby.

DISORDERS OF HANDS, FEET, NAILS, HAIR AND BREASTS

Bunion (Hallux Valgus) An outward displacement of the distal end of the first metatarsal, covered by a thickened skin.

Corn A localised thickening of the epidermis. It may be on top of or underneath the foot. It is due to continual pressure on the area.

Soft Corn This is a type of corn occurring between the toes, which is moist and soft.

Callus A general thickening of the epidermis due to pressure or friction on either the hands or feet.

Hard Skin An exceptional build-up of thickened epidermal cells often found under the foot. Due to lack of care to rubbing of ill-fitting shoes.

Hammertoes A permanent bending of the toes making them look like small hammers. It may affect just one or all the toes. Caused by wearing shoes that are too small, especially in childhood.

Onychia An inflammation affecting the nail bed.

Hangnail A splitting of the cuticle at the side or the base of the nail. It is usually caused by excessive dryness or poor hand care.

Whitlow An acute inflammation of deep-seated tissues of the fingers, causing an abcess. This may need medical attention.

Ingrowing Nail The nail extends sidways into the nail wall. It is often caused by poor-fitting shoes or a lack of foot care.

Longitudinal Ridges See page 128. These may be caused by illness or poor diet (a lack of calcium or iron), damage to the matrix or lack of nail care.

Transverse Ridges See page 127. These may be due to temporary poor health or they may be hereditary.

Flaking and Splitting Nails See pages 128-9. These may be caused by poor diet or frequent washing in hot water and detergent.

Spoon-Shaped Nails See page 128. These may indicate anaemia in some cases, especially in middle-aged women.

Excessively Curved Nails These may be found in some cases of congenital heart conditions.

White Spots in the Nail These may be caused by a blow to the nail or matrix.

Bruised Nail This may show as a dark discoloured spot under the nail.

Dry and Brittle Nails This is often caused by poor diet or illness or be due to rough filing.

Fungus This forms dull, yellow patches around the nail. It is highly infectious.

Ringworm This forms a yellowish mass around the nail. The nail becomes spongy and may separate from the nail bed.

Athletes Foot A fungal infection usually affecting the foot. Itching and sodden white skin may appear between the toes. It may develop cracks and fissures as well as small watery blisters. It is highly infectious.

Psoriasis This can affect any skin surface. It may affect the nail bed, nail wall or cause 'pitting' of the nail plate. It looks like flaky, silvery scales and sometimes has a red ring around the edge. It may also affect the scalp where the scales can tend to build up.

Warts These are small swellings in the skin caused by a virus. Some have a rough, horny surface; others may be pearly smooth. They may be light or dark in colour. They may be formed in clusters or singly. They can easily be contracted from an infected person or by self-infection.

The most common types of wart are:

Verruca Vulgaris (common wart) This is a dark, raised wart found mainly on the hands and sometimes on the face.

Verruca Plana (flat wart) This is small and usually found on the face and hands.

Verruca Plantaris This is usually found on the soles of the foot. It is flattened due to pressure and may cause discomfort or even pain.

Arthritis Inflammation of the joints, causing pain and swelling.

Alopecia Areata Partial hair loss, particularly of the scalp. This condition is more common in the male.

Dandruff The scalp gives off flakes or epidermal cells, which appear as white flakes, and accumulate on the scalp. There may be irritation.

Seborrhoea A scaling and redness of the scalp caused by a disorder of the sebaceous glands. In severe cases it may produce excessive sebum accompanied by pustules.

Mastitis Inflammation of breast tissue. It is most common during the first two months of breast-feeding a baby. If left untreated it can lead to an abscess.

Breast Tumour These may be simple cysts or adenoma or they may be carcinogenic. If diagnosed early this form of cancer can usually be completely eradicated.

PART B

Treatments

There are many different treatments that a therapist can perform for clients, and there are a number of ways that these treatments may be carried out. Some of them are described in the following chapters. Teachers and other therapists may perform them in different ways. The therapist must always be guided by the manufacturer's instructions when using instruments or special preparations.

Chapter 10

Skin Analysis and Cleansing

It is claimed by some authorities, including even a few doctors, that cleansing the skin is of no benefit other than for social reasons. While this may be so, most of us will agree that a clean skin certainly looks more healthy and attractive.

Dead cells are continually being shed by the skin. Dust particles, natural secretions from the sebaceous and sweat glands and stale make-up all combine to block the pores. This can create spots and black-heads, giving the skin a dull appearance.

Cleansing is the most important procedure that the therapist will ever learn. As the waste matter and surplus oils are gently removed, the skin will start to look fresher. It will be able to function more effectively. However it is very important that the therapist knows what type of skin is being worked on.

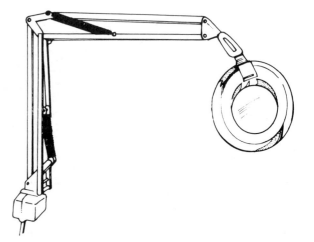

A cold light magnifier

SKIN ANALYSIS

For the sake of convenience the skin is generally divided into four main types: *normal, dry, oily* and *combination*.

The skin is a living organ. It can vary from season to season or even from week to week depending upon the general health of the person as well as external factors. These can include the atmosphere in the place of work or home environment, the sort of diet followed, or hormonal balance. The life style should be examined to see if there is sufficient exercise, relaxation and sleep. The client should be asked if they take proper care of their skin.

In order to ascertain what skin type a person has, the therapist should thoroughly cleanse the skin. It should then be examined using a strong light and, if possible, a magnifying glass.

SKIN COLOUR

The first thing to note is the colour of the skin. This is not just black, brown, yellow or white. There are many varying tones. Black and brown skin has more melanin present than yellow or white skin. People who live and work out of doors in all weather, especially bright sunlight, have a darker coloured skin than is normally associated with their ethnic background. Those people who spend much of their lives out of the natural sunlight, such as night workers, may have a paler and thinner skin than would normally be expected.

Some skins may appear to have a pink or ruddy complexion. This is due to the number of superficial blood vessels showing through. Other skin colourings include olive or yellow tinges, which could be due to the amount of carotene or even bile pigment present. The ethnic background of the client must always be considered. Other factors that can affect the skin tone include certain drugs, illness or artificial tanning lotions.

SKIN TYPES

Normal Skin

This type of skin has a fine, even texture. It has a good balance of moisture and oil secretion. The blood circulation is good, so the skin looks clear with a rosy hue (white skin) or mauve hue (black skin). It should feel warm to the touch. The texture is neither too thick nor too thin. There are no open pores or greasy areas and spots or blemishes rarely develop. It should have no dry, flaky patches and little sign of lining.

Dry Skin

This condition is caused by an insufficient secretion of sebum. It has a fine texture and no visible pores. It may have a thin, almost transparent look. It can look and often feel tight, but will show lines and wrinkles, particularly around the eyes and mouth, from quite an early age. It is often sensitive, and likely to develop broken capillaries. It can react strongly to both internal and external influences.

Sensitive Skin

This skin is usually dry with fine pores. There may be broken capillaries over the cheeks and nose. There may also be a few comedones. It may react to heat, cold, pressure, irritation or nervous conditions. It often responds to an allergic stimulus.

Allergic Skin

Any type of skin may produce an allergic reaction to either internal or external stimulus. It is, however, more prevalent in the dry skin conditions.

Mature Skin

This skin is dry, due to insufficient moisture and sebum. Premature lines lie around the eyes and mouth as well as across the forehead. Skin tone is reduced as elasticity is lessened. The skin may be loose due to the loss of the subcutaneous fat. Blood supply may be poor, which could result in blemishes.

Dehydrated Skin

This can be identified by its extreme dryness. It may appear to be tight. It may be dull or pale due to a poor circulation and have a fine 'orange peel' appearance.

Oily Skin

This condition is caused by an over-secretion of the sebaceous glands. The skin surface may be uneven, having large open pores, comedones or even pustules. Poor circulation may make it look sallow with a shiny or greasy appearance.

Seborrhoeic Skin

There are two kinds of seborrhoea: *seborrhoea sicca* and *seborrhoea oleosa*.

Seborrhoea sicca is a dry form of the condition. The dead epidermal cells mix with the excess sebaceous oils to form large flakes, which fall from the skin and scalp. This gives the appearance of dryness.

In *seborrhoea oleosa*, the sebaceous glands excrete far more sebum than is needed by the skin. The skin looks very oily and shiny as does the scalp and hair.

Often both conditions are present. The pores are enlarged, there are comedones and often pustules, and there may also be scarring. The circulation is poor, giving rise to a sallow complexion. Often this condition can lead to acne.

Oedematous Skin

In this condition the skin looks swollen and puffy. If it is depressed with the fingertips it remains white rather than springing back to its normal form and colour. It is caused by poor circulation and weak lymphatic drainage. It may also occur when there is too much salt in the diet, during the premenstrual time or where tissues are damaged.

Combination Skin

This type of skin is made up of both oily and dry skin. The oily skin often, but not always, forms a 'T' zone across the forehead and down the nose and chin. There may be enlarged pores on the upper and inner parts of the cheeks and nose. The skin on the rest of the face and neck is dry, even flaky.

There are two forms of combination skin: oily/normal combination skin and dry/normal combination skin. In oily/normal combination skin, the centre panel is oily while the rest of the skin is of a normal type. In the dry/normal combination skin, the centre panel may be normal while there are dry areas on the cheeks.

Diagnosis of Skin Types using a Wood's Lamp

Certain skin types and conditions show up more easily under the light from a Wood's lamp.

A Wood's lamp gives off deep ultraviolet rays. It must be used in a completely dark room to get the best effect.

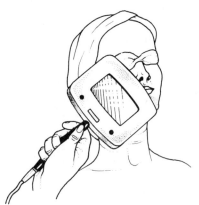

A Wood's lamp

Various skin conditions show as different shades:

1 Normal skin shows through as a blue-white.
2 Oily skin shows as a yellowish-pink.
3 Dry skin shows as a light violet.
4 Dehydrated skin shows as purple.
5 Thick skin – the thicker the skin, the whiter the fluorescence.
6 Thin skin – the thinner the skin, the more purple the fluorescence.
7 Areas of pigmentation show up brown.
8 Dead skin cells show as white spots.

COMMON ALLERGIES

An allergy is the body's reaction to a 'foreign' substance. The skin reacts in several ways. There may be heat, redness, itching and irritation. This may be followed by swelling, vesicles and crusty sores.

Allergies result from four main causes: *inhalants*, *contacts*, *ingestants* and *infection*.

Inhalants
Tree, grass and flower pollen, and perfume are among the things that can cause hay fever. The effects can be blocked sinuses (causing pain and headaches), sneezing and running eyes. The skin may become oedematous and tender.

Contacts
Dust, animal fur, fabrics, plants and cosmetics are among some of the common allergens. They may cause some of the same symptoms as in hay fever or an eczema.

Ingestants
Certain foods and drinks such as strawberries or shell fish may produce urticaria (see page 29).

Infection
Medical infection, insect stings and bites may cause both a local swelling or a general oedema.

Sometimes a particular cosmetic product is suspected of being an allergen. The simplest way to diagnose an allergy is to ask the client to stop using that particular product for a couple of weeks. If the symptoms clear up, this may have been the cause of the problem. It could, of course, have been produced by something quite different. If the client wishes to continue with the same product, she can then start to re-use it. If, however, the symptoms return she should be advised against using it again.

In cosmetics, very often the allergies are caused by a particular colour, perfume compound or chemical used in one item of a manufacturer's range. It may be just one lipstick, nail polish or perfume. Other items in the same range would probably not have any adverse effect.

SKIN CLEANSING

Cleansing is a very important procedure. The purpose is to remove dead skin cells, dust and grime, and stale make-up. Only when the skin is thoroughly cleansed can other treatments be performed.

A good therapist may like to use this time to talk to the client. Explain how cleansing can be carried out by the client each day at home following the same gentle movements used by the therapist.

No matter what the treatment, any movements on the skin must be gentle and controlled. Heavy handling will stretch the skin, cause broken capillaries and over-stimulate the sebaceous glands. It will damage the skin texture and also be uncomfortable for the client.

There are many methods of cleansing. Each tutor has a favourite method, and no doubt students adopt their own styles before too long.

One school of thought recommends spreading the cleansing milk or cream over the face and neck and then removing either with pads of damp cotton-wool or blotting off with a tissue. Others apply the cleanser to damp cotton-wool pads and wipe them over the face.

Preparation

The therapist should have everything ready before commencing the treatment. It wastes time not to do this, and a client who is kept waiting may soon become irritated.

Ask the client to remove her outer clothing and any jewellery that she is wearing. She may wish to put on a strapless gown or just wrap a towel around herself. Then help her onto the couch or chair and put warm towels or a blanket over her. In warm weather or in hot countries a cooling fan will be appreciated.

Requirements

Creams and Lotions
Cleansing cream
Cleansing milk
Eye make-up remover
Skin tonic
Antiseptic
Mask
Moisturiser

Utensils
Cotton buds
Damp cotton-wool pads
Tissues
Spatulae
Orange sticks
Eyebrow forceps
Comedone extractor

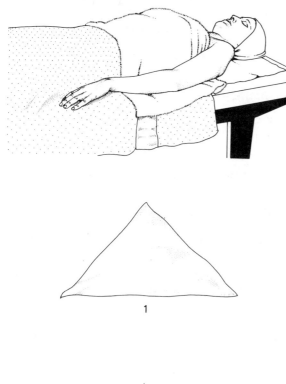

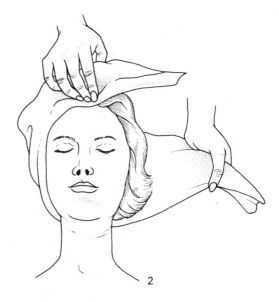

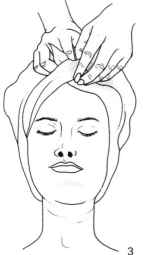

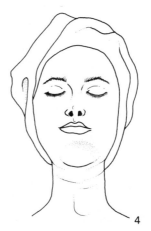

Applying a head towel

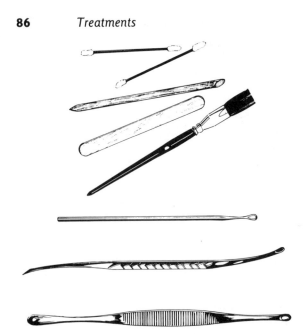

Mask brush
Bowl for cotton-wool
Bowl for mask water
Receiver for used equipment
Receiver for waste materials
Head band, triangle or hat
Gown

Equipment
  Couch or chair
  Trolley

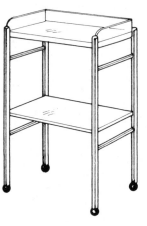

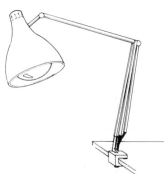

Infra-red lamp

Infra-red lamp or steamer
Magnifying lamp for inspection
Wood's lamp
Couch covers
Couch paper
Covering towels or blankets
Gown for clients
Stool (for therapist)

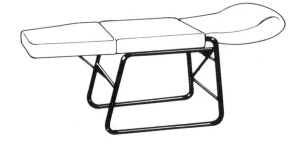

Cleansing the Eyes

The eyes are usually cleansed before the rest of the face so as not to spread any make-up to the rest of the skin. Cleanse each eye separately.

There are two different ways to clean the eyes:

Method A
1 Apply cleansing milk or eye make-up gel lightly with the fingertips. Use a circular movement all around the eyes and over the eyelids.
2 Remove the cleansing medium with pads of damp cotton-wool. Lift the eyebrow with the fingertips of one hand. Use downward movements with the cotton-wool pad over the eyelid and lashes. Then gently wipe the pad outwards over the upper

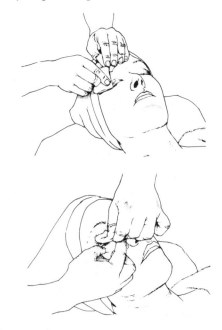

eyelid area. Finally wipe outwards under the lower lid. Rotate the pad so that a clean part of it is always used. The eyes are wiped with an outward movement so that no 'foreign' matter is pushed into the tear duct.

3 Repeat the procedure until the eye area is clean.
4 Repeat on the other eye. Do not use the same piece of cotton-wool on the second eye.

Method B

1 Place a thin cotton-wool pad under the lower lashes of one eye. Dip both ends of a cotton bud into cleansing milk or eye make-up remover.
2 Gently lift the skin above one eye at the eyebrow. Lightly rotate the cotton bud down the eyelid and lashes and over the cotton-wool pad. Repeat until the area is clean.
3 Wipe the eyelid with damp cotton-wool, from the inside corner to the outside.
4 Repeat on the second eye.
5 Remove the lower pad.

Cleansing the Lips

These are also cleansed before the rest of the face. Spread cleansing milk onto two pads of cotton-wool. Hold one pad at each corner of the mouth. Lift one hand and place it at the other side of the mouth. Gently slide it back to its original position. Repeat with the other hand. Repeat this procedure, turning the cotton-wool around until the mouth is clean. Blot gently with a tissue to remove any surplus oils.

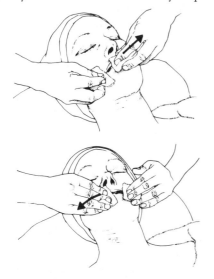

Cleansing the Face

There are two methods of performing this procedure. There are, however, a number of different patterns used to work over the parts of the face.

All the patterns follow a similar basic sequence such as:

1 neck
2 chin
3 cheeks
4 nose
5 forehead.

Method A

1 Apply sufficient cleansing milk or cleansing cream all over the client's face. Use the pads of the fingertips to perform either circular or stroking movements as appropriate to each area. Some people like to work on one side of the face at a time. Others prefer to work with both hands moving over both sides of the face simultaneously. A third group prefers to use a combination of both methods.

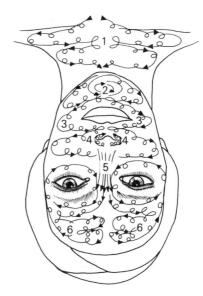

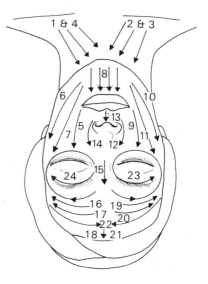

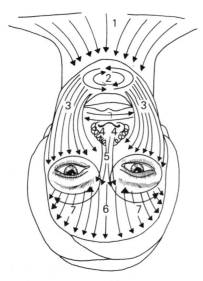

2 Remove the cleansing milk or cleansing cream with a damp pad of cotton-wool in each hand, again following a set pattern. Turn or change the cotton-wool pads frequently until all the cleanser is removed. Repeat the procedure until the skin is clean. Two cleanses are usually sufficient.

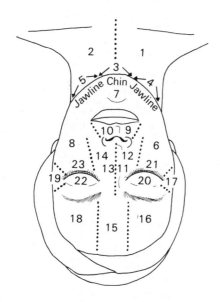

It is important to use sufficient cleanser so that the cotton-wool can be smoothly moved over the skin without dragging it. The action must be gentle and even, with no harsh or sudden movements.

Method B

1 Apply cleansing milk to two pads of cotton-wool. Have one pad in each hand.
2 Follow the same pattern used for the removal of cleanser in method A.

Toning

When the skin is thoroughly clean, apply skin tonic to two damp pads of cotton-wool. Follow the set pattern for cleansing. Repeat the toning a second time.

Moisturising

If no further treatment is to be given, apply a moisturiser, smoothing it all over the face and neck. Use an effleurage-type movement (page 94) to aid penetration. Blot off any surplus.

Blotting

There are several methods for blotting the face:

Method A

1 Make a hole in the centre of a tissue. Place the tissue over the face. Have the nose showing through the hole.
2 Fold the tissue down over the face, section by section, blotting the skin as you do so.

Method B

1 Spread a folded tissue across the forehead. Smooth one hand across it to blot the face dry.
2 Peel the tissue off and place it over half the face. Smooth gently around the eye, nose and mouth and across the cheek.
3 Place the tissue on the other cheek and repeat.
4 Place the tissue over the chin and neck and smooth dry. This method may take longer but because the client can always see out of one eye, it does not feel 'claustrophobic'.

The skin is now ready for inspection under a magnifying or Wood's lamp or for whatever treatment is to follow.

FACE MASKS

A mask may be used for several reasons: to remove dead skin cells; to stimulate and refine the skin; or to soothe or nourish, depending on its type or the ingredients. It may be applied after cleansing but before any treatment, or at the end of a treatment.

The mask should always be removed from the jar or bowl with a spatula. It should then be applied with a clean, damp brush.

The mask must be applied quickly and evenly to the face and neck. Avoid putting it on the delicate skin around the eyes, in the nostrils or the mouth. Some people find it easier to start at the throat while others prefer to start at the forehead.

Where the skin is extra fine or sensitive, the mask may be applied very thinly. It may be removed from the cheeks as soon as the rest of the mask is applied. In some instances it may be omitted from these areas altogether.

Where there are areas of congestion or spots, some people may wish to apply an extra thick layer of mask. If the skin is a combination type, you can apply more than one mask at a time.

A mask should be applied to one area at a time. It should be applied in sequence, e.g.

1 around the neck
2 the chin
3 one cheek, then the other cheek
4 the nose
5 the forehead.

Apply cool eye pads if the client wishes to have them.

The mask may be left on for 5–20 minutes. The time depends upon the sensitivity of the skin, the comfort of the client, the type of mask used and the external temperature.

The mask should be removed with cotton-wool pads rinsed in luke-warm water. Care should be taken so as not to get water into the client's eyes, nose or mouth. Disposable cotton-wool is more hygienic than sponges which are difficult to sterilise thoroughly.

For details of masks see Chapter 17.

Contra-indications

A mask should not be used on people prone to allergic reactions, or over the following conditions:
    sensitive areas of skin
    recent scar tissue
    areas of broken capillaries
    high vascular diffusion
    infectious skin conditions.

THE LONDON CLEANSE

This simple cleansing treatment was devised by the author and is a favourite with her students at Wendover House College, London. It can be easily adapted to suit many skin conditions, from the congested type to acne.

Method

1 Cleanse the face very thoroughly with cleansing milk.
2 Apply skin tonic.

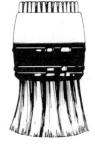

3 Apply a skin shampoo with a soft, damp brush or sponge. Use gentle circular movements all over the face and neck for 1–3 minutes. Avoid the delicate tissues around the eyes, nostrils and mouth. If the skin is rubbed hard or for too long it is likely to peel or become sore.
4 Blot the skin dry with a tissue.
5 Wipe over the area at least twice with tonic of a high acidic content until the soapy action of the shampoo has ceased.
6 'Open' the pores by using steam or an infra-red lamp for approximately five minutes. Protect the eyes while doing so.
7 Use a comedone extractor to remove any comedones, trapped sebum or pustules.
8 Wipe the area with a strong antiseptic solution.
9 Apply a heavy emollient cream.
10 Apply direct high frequency (pages 122–4) for up to five minutes, 'sparking' over the worst affected areas.
11 Blot the face and then apply skin tonic to remove the cream.
12 Apply a soft mask and leave on for 7–15 minutes according to the skin condition. Remove with cotton-wool pads and warm water.
13 Apply a final skin tonic and blot dry.
14 Apply a moisturiser.
15 As with all treatments, recommend that no make-up be used for a few hours.

EXFOLIATION

This treatment removes the outer layer of the epidermis and any dead cells. Either a solution or a cream may be used. It may be of vegetable or chemical origin. It will soften the dead keratinised cells so that they may be gently removed. A cream may sometimes contain such ingredients as crushed nuts or pumice. The amount of skin and dead cells removed depends on the process employed.

The treatment may result in redness and in some cases, pigmentation. This is because the blood flow is stimulated towards the surface. The client should be warned that the iron content of the blood can be affected by ultraviolet lamps, natural sunlight or a hormone-based medicine. It can produce a brown pigment for up to six months after some treatments. In most people there is little or no reaction.

Exfoliation can be performed in several ways:
a mask
vegetable peeling
chemical (progressive) peeling
abrasion.

Exfoliation Mask

There are several forms of this simple basic treatment, both for the professional to use and as retail packs for the client to use. Usually it is a cream mask base containing a granular substance such as nut kernels, husks or pumice.

Method

1 Cleanse, tone and warm the skin in the usual manner.
2 Apply the mask. Sometimes an infra-red lamp is placed over the face to speed up the drying process.
3 Gently rub off the mask using a light circular action of the fingertips. If the mask has dried too firmly, it may be dampened with warm water or a spray.
4 Any remaining mask may be removed with cotton-wool pads, again using a circular movement.
5 When the skin is quite clean, blot dry and apply a moisturiser.

Always follow the manufacturer's instructions.

Vegetable Peeling

This is a rejuvenating treatment for dry or lined skin. There are a number of proprietary biological peeling agents on the market using many different ingredients. A course of ten treatments should be given. They should be performed two or three times a week over a three to four week period.

Contra-indications

Infected skin (vesicles, pustules etc.)
Irritated skin
Abrasions
Hypersensitive skin (treat with extra caution)
High vascular tones and broken capillaries

Method

1 Cleanse the skin with cleansing milk and tonic.
2 Remove all trace of oils. Use surgical spirit if necessary.

3 Warm the skin using either an infra-red lamp or steam.
4 Apply a softening lotion to the dry skin. Use a tapotement movement (page 95) for 3–5 minutes or until it has all been absorbed to pat the lotion onto the skin.
5 Apply a cream mask, avoiding the eyes, nostrils and mouth.
6 Place eye pads over the eyes and allow the client to rest for fifteen minutes.

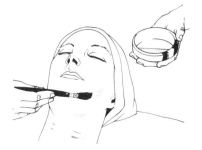

7 Use a light circular movement to remove the mask. Take it off with warm water and cotton-wool pads.
8 Blot the skin dry.
9 Massage the skin with a hydrating cream for 20 minutes.
10 Remove any excess cream with damp cotton-wool pads. Leave sufficient cream on the face to act as a moisturiser.
11 Advise the client that make-up should not be used for several hours.

There are many different types of skin peeling. The therapist should read the manufacturer's instructions carefully before proceeding with this treatment.

Progressive Chemical Peeling

This treatment is suitable for lessening the effect of coarse, open pores, post-acne scarring, greasy, sallow or discoloured skin. It is very useful for removing the remains of a suntan.

The treatment helps to clear the skin but does not get rid of acne scars. It is, however, quite a harsh treatment and can cause skin irritation. The therapist must have a good knowledge of the skin and how it will react to chemicals. It is often advisable to perform a patch test.

The active ingredients are often resorcinol or salicylic acid though there are several other agents. Treatments should usually be given three times a week on alternate days, in a course usually consisting of ten treatments. For a mild peeling, the treatments may be given at weekly intervals.

The powder may come in five graduated strengths. The treatments usually commence with the weakest powder (no. 1). The strength is increased on alternate treatments if there is no adverse reaction.

Contra-indications

Infected skin (vesicles, pustules etc.)
Irritated skin
Abrasions
Sensitive skin/broken capillaries
Dehydrated skin
Mature skin
Fine skin

Method

1 Cleanse the skin with cleansing milk and skin tonic.
2 Remove all trace of oils with a spirit solution.
3 'Open' the pores using an infra-red lamp or steam for five minutes.
4 Apply an oil to the delicate tissue under the eyes.
5 Mix the appropriately numbered powder with the 'active' lotion to form a thin paste.
6 Use a brush to spread the paste evenly over the face, and the neck if required.
7 Avoid the delicate skin around the eyes, the nostrils and the mouth and any skin lesions.
8 Leave on for 5–15 minutes depending on the client's skin reaction. If a strong irritation is felt, remove the mask at once. If there is no reaction, increase the time by two minutes on the next visit and on alternate treatments.
    Note on the client's record card what number powder was used and how long it was left on for. If an adverse reaction occurs, note this down and do not increase the strength of the powder for the next treatment. Decrease the time the paste is left on the skin.
9 Remove the paste by sponging off with warm water.
10 Dry the skin thoroughly.
11 Apply a hydrating cream and massage the face for ten minutes using extractive movements (pinching, tapotement etc.).
12 Remove the surplus cream by blotting with a tissue. Clean the skin with skin tonic, and dry thoroughly.
13 As with any treatment, the therapist should recommend that no make-up is used for several hours.

Always be sure to follow the manufacturer's instructions.

Progressive Peeling to Lighten Dark Skin

1 Clean the skin with cleansing milk, skin tonic and then a spirit solution.
2 'Open' the pores using an infra-red lamp or steam.
3 Apply oil to the delicate skin under the eyes.
4 Commence the course of treatments with a medium strength powder (no. 3).
5 Wait until it is very dry before removing it with a wet cotton-wool pad, using circular movements all over the face.
6 Freshen the skin with rose water or camomile lotion.
7 On the days that the client is not receiving a treatment she should apply a hydrating cream and massage her face for a quarter of an hour. The cream is then removed with skin tonic.

It must be emphasised that no other cream or oil should be used for the duration of a progressive peeling treatment.

Brush Cleansing

The skin may be cleansed with a light brush and a liquid cleanser, using a circular movement with light pressure to remove dead skin cells. The movement must be very light or too much of the epidermis will be removed, causing pain or even abrasions. The brushes may be electrical, battery operated or manual. Some brush sets on the market contain an abrasive pad of pumice. These are far too harsh to use on the face.

Abrasion

This is a method for removing part of the epidermis by means of stiff fibre or metal brushes or grinding disks revolving at high speed. It is a very delicate operation performed by plastic surgeons where the skin has been badly pitted by acne or where there are scars or deep lines. Some therapy machines also have such brushes. At no time should the therapist try to perform this operation.

A SPANISH FACIAL

This special facial treatment has been compiled with the assistance of Mrs Christine Campbell-Salisbury, founder of the Marbella Hair and Beauty College in Spain.

Spain is a place of blue sky and sunshine. In the valleys there drifts the heady aroma of orange blossom. People who live in this sunny climate may unfortunately suffer from dry skin and require an extra special treatment. The Spanish facial is such a treatment.

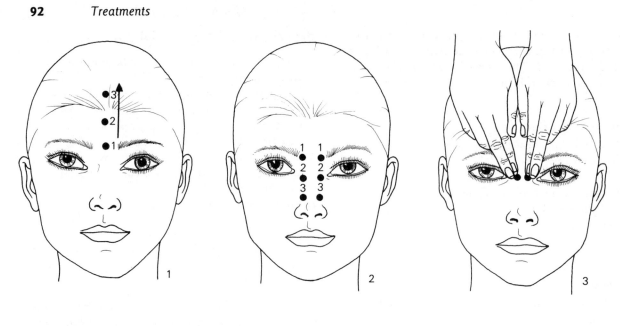

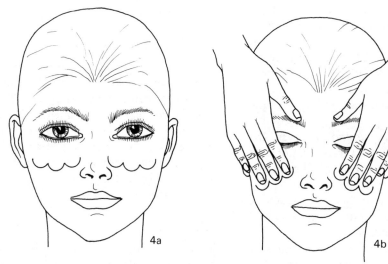

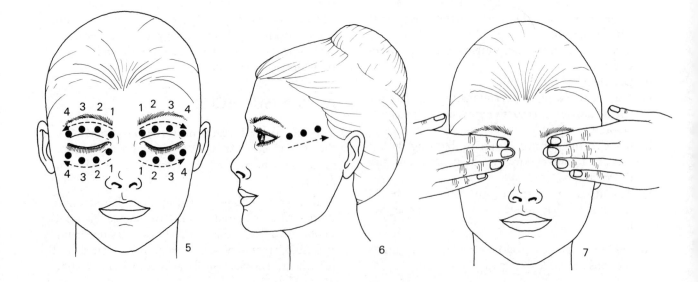

Method

1 Cleanse the face with a mild cleansing milk.
2 Prepare a mild skin peel with a dash of orange flower water.
3 Massage the skin with an enriched hydrating cream to replenish the lost oils.
4 Steam the face without using ozone. Use orange essence in the water.
5 Perform iontophoresis (pages 115–6) using a super-hydrating ampoule or gel.
6 Apply a gentle chamomile-based emollient mask.
7 Prepare water for a compress in a pretty bowl. Add two drops of orange oil and a couple of ice cubes.
8 Take six tissues and fold them into strips. Immerse them in the water, then squeeze out the excess water.
9 Apply the strips to the face, starting at the base of the neck and work up the face. Mould them gently into the contours of the face to form a mask.
10 Apply gentle pressure to the shiatsu points (opposite).
11 Peel off the paper mask.
12 Finish the treatment by giving your client a glass of fresh orange juice, spiked with mint.

AN AFRICAN FACIAL SEQUENCE

This treatment sequence has been devised by Mrs Vera Roper, founder of the Afrodite School in Nairobi, Kenya.

The treatment uses products from the Dead Sea. It is particularly suitable for teenage *acne vulgaris*. It has been noted that the dark scars which usually remain following this disorder have faded to their normal skin colour. This treatment also provides a safe and natural alternative to skin lightening products.

Method

1 Cleanse the eyes and lips using a mild cleanser and toner.
2 Lightly apply a hydrophilic cleansing oil over the face and neck. Avoid the eyes and lips.
3 Gradually add drops of warm water to the oil. Work up to an emulsion with the fingertips.
4 Massage lightly with a circular movement until the face and neck have been thoroughly cleaned.
5 Blot with a tissue to absorb all the oil.

6 Remove the residue with warm water, then apply a toner.
7 Spread a treatment cream containing active minerals fairly thickly over the area to be treated.
8 Apply the activating crystals sparingly onto the cream.
9 Lightly work the crystals into the cream until the reaction is observed, i.e. the combined products change into a liquid.
10 Place cotton-wool pads over the eyes. Leave the liquid on the face for up to ten minutes. *Caution*: if any tingling is experienced or an erythema (page 26) occurs, remove the liquid thoroughly and cool the skin with a compress. This reaction denotes that this skin is too sensitive to continue with the treatment.
11 Blot off any remaining liquid.
12 Rinse the skin thoroughly with warm water to neutralise it. A skin tonic should be applied.
13 Apply eye pads. Apply a cold water compress to the area and leave for ten minutes.
14 Blot the skin dry and then apply a thin layer of the active treatment cream.
15 Mix the mask powder with the gel and apply over the cream, leaving the eyes and lips free. Make sure that the mask is thick at the edges.
16 Remove the mask when it has just set by 'flapping up' at the lower edge. Peel it slowly upwards. If correctly applied, the mask will be removed in one piece.
17 Apply a toner containing special minerals.
18 Blot the skin dry. On examination, the skin should be soft, refined and two or three shades lighter, nearer to the tone of the skin on the body.
19 Give the client a mirror and ask her to watch carefully as the sun barrier is applied. Impress upon her the importance of its regular daily use.
20 Dot a small amount of the sun barrier over the face and neck. Lightly blend all over the face and neck so as to protect against the ultraviolet rays of the sun.
21 Explain to the client that the ultraviolet rays of the sun can damage, age and darken the skin. An ultraviolet barrier cream containing ingredients to filter out both the ultraviolet A and B rays must be used to protect the skin from burning and darkening.

Make sure that the client fully understands how to use all the preparations that she will need to purchase to use at home. Stress that the products must not be used near the eyes or on the mouth.

Chapter 11

Facial Massage

Facial massage is probably the most frequently performed of all the treatments. It is the one treatment when the therapist has actual contact with the client. The therapist's hands must be kept soft and flexible, in order to regulate the pressure while working over the different tissues. An even rhythm must be maintained with no sudden or jerking movements. The therapist must develop an acute sense of touch and awareness so that just the right pressure can be used in order to both stimulate and relax the tissues.

A facial massage should be performed in a quiet, relaxed atmosphere. A therapist should never give the impression of being rushed while performing a facial massage. The therapist should base the massage movements on the requirements of the client, such as the condition of the skin, muscular tone, vascular condition and the nervous state of the client.

MASSAGE EFFECTS

The purpose of a facial massage is to improve the skin condition by breaking down toxins and assisting their removal by stimulating the circulation and lymphatic systems. It also assists the blood supply to bring nourishment to the skin and muscle fibres in the form of oxygen, proteins etc. Certain movements will stimulate or calm the nerve endings thereby assisting them to become more receptive to sensation. Often movements will have a tonic effect on the muscles. Some movements will have a general relaxing effect. Any tension in the neck or shoulders will be eased. A facial massage should relax the client and produce a feeling of well-being. The client should both look and feel better for the experience.

Contra-indications
  Broken capillaries
  Infected areas (pustules, cold sores etc.)
  Recent scar tissue
  Swollen or oedematous areas
  Painful areas (such as over a toothache)
  Medical conditions such as Bell's palsy

Several types of medium are suitable for facial massage. One of the most popular is a cold cream, but a light massage oil may be preferred. Care must be taken to see that it does not run too freely. The most pleasurable effects can be obtained with the use of an aromatherapy oil.

MASSAGE TECHNIQUES

There are a number of basic movements for facial massage. Each tutor will have her own special techniques. A good therapist will build on them and adapt them to suit the individual client.

The different movements include:

Effleurage
Effleurage may be used over the face, chest, shoulders and neck. It may be performed with the palms of the hands. On the face it is usually performed with the pads of the fingers as well as the palms. The actual tips of the fingers are never used in effleurage.

Effleurage is a slow, rhythmic stroking movement. It is always used at the beginning of the massage. The purpose of this is to spread the oil or cream, to allow the client to get used to the therapist's hands moving over the face, to enable the therapist to feel the contours of the client's face and to note any reaction to the movement.

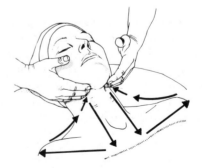

An effleurage may be used after more stimulating movements both to calm and relax the client. It may also be used for lymphatic drainage.

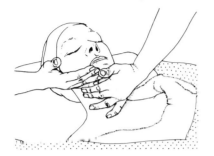

Petrissage

Petrissage helps to break down and eliminate waste products. It is performed with the ball of the finger, not the tip. Occasionally the ball of the thumb may be used. It is a circular movement using pressure on soft tissue lying over bone. The finger must not slide over the skin but move the tissue over the bone.

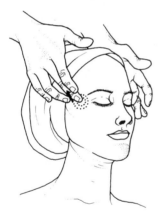

Pinchment

The skin is picked up between the fingers and thumb in a series of light pinches and then released. The rhythmic movement has a stimulating effect as well as being extractive.

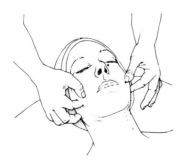

Friction

This is also a form of petrissage. These are small movements performed with the finger pads. They may be performed in a circular manner or straight as in a scissor movement.

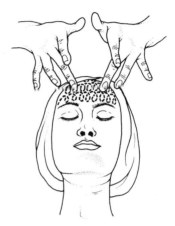

Circular friction

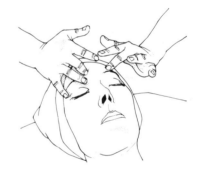

Scissor friction

Tapotement

Tapotement is a quick, light percussive movement using the pads of the fingers. It is used to increase the blood supply to the areas, to increase muscle tone and lessen nervous tension. The rhythm and touch must be even or it will irritate the client.

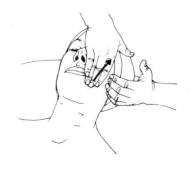

Tapping

This is a form of tapotement. The pads of the fingers are used together, in a light tapping movement along the jawline and on the buccinator muscles. Sometimes the palms of the hands may also be used to create a vacuum across the cheeks.

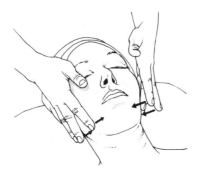

Another form of tapotement is the *butterfly* movement. In this all the fingertips are 'played' independently, as though practising piano scales. The movement is very light, hence the term 'butterfly'.

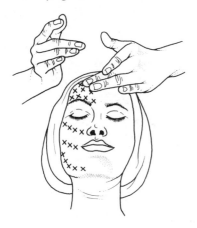

Vibrations

This is a fine, trembling movement using the fingers or the whole of the hand. The movement may be *static*, that is, remaining in one place or *running*, where the fingers travel over an area. It has both a stimulating and a relaxing effect on the tissues.

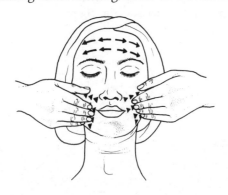

Stroking

This is a form of effleurage. It is often performed on the forehead. Stroking may be performed with the palms of the hand alternately stroking up the frontalis.

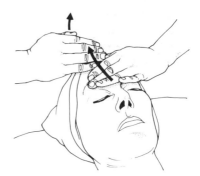

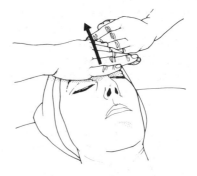

Stroking may also be performed by using two hands alternately, trailing the one whole hand across the forehead while the other hand holds the temple to stop the head rolling over.

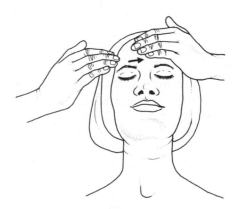

Sliding

This is a drainage movement performed on the cheeks, draining from the nose out towards the preauricular lymphatic node.

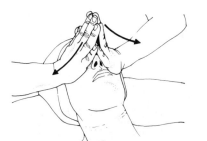

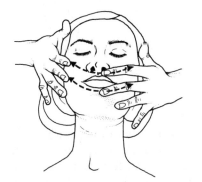

Eye Circling

Any movement performed near the eyes must be very light and gentle. Eye movements may be performed in a gliding, circling or tapping manner.

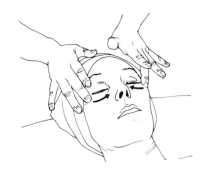

Gliding

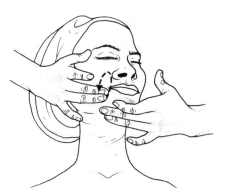

Cheek Movements

Other cheek movements include tapping and circling.

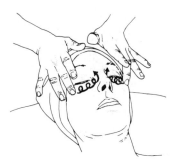

Circling

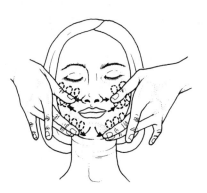

Cheek tapping

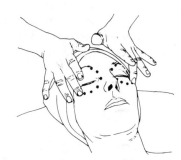

Tapping

Cheek circling

Nose Movements

Care must be taken when working on the nose to ensure that the nostrils are not constricted.

One movement is that of sliding the fingertips lightly down the nose.

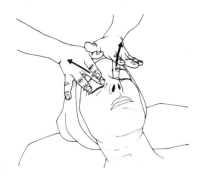

A circular movement may also be performed around the mouth.

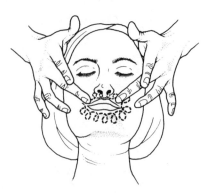

Alternatively, small, circular movements may be performed with the fingertips around the nose and across the cheeks.

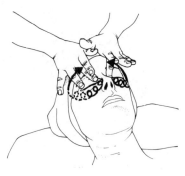

Knuckling

This movement is performed with the knuckles of the fingers rotating over an area. It may be performed very lightly over the lower cheeks and sides of the neck. A little more pressure may be applied over the chest area. A firm pressure may be applied to the back of the neck and shoulders. The main purpose is to break down waste matter in the underlying muscular tissue.

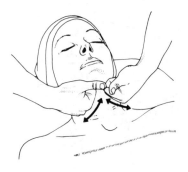

Mouth Movements

This is a sliding action, using two fingers of one hand to slide back across the mouth while holding the corner of the mouth with the other hand. A lifting action at the corners of the mouth should be performed after each slide.

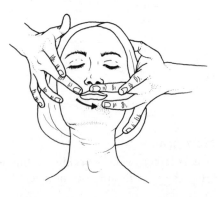

Kneading

This is performed rather like a petrissage with the fingertips on the neck. Superficial tissue is picked up and rolled against firmer tissue lying underneath.

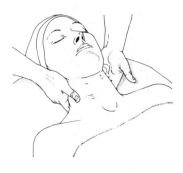

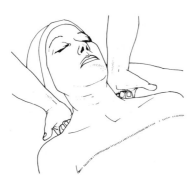

When kneading is performed on the face it must be very gentle, like a soft wringing movement.

Chin and Throat Movements
These include gliding and tapping along the jaw line.

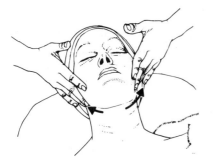

Gliding

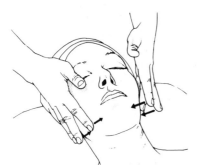

Tapping

Stroking up the throat may be followed by circling.

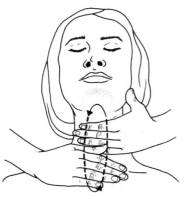

Stroking

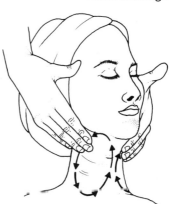

Circling

Pressure Movements
Pressure may be applied to certain points of the neck, face and head. They may be on shiatsu points or motor points. The pressure is usually applied with the ball of the third finger. It is held for four seconds.

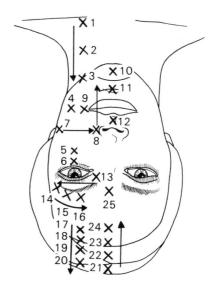

Pressure points

Neck Movements
Movements on the neck may include effleurage, tapotement, pinchment, knuckling, kneading and gliding. Petrissage may be performed up the cervical spine.

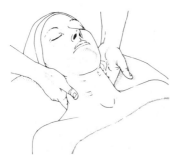

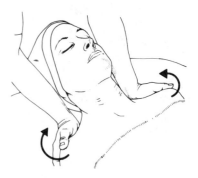

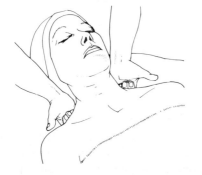

Chest Movements

Movements on the front of the chest include a deep, sweeping effleurage, kneading and petrissage. Movements on the back of the chest include kneading on the trapezius and deltoid muscles. Deep-breathing exercises may also be included.

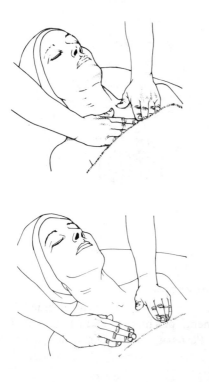

A JAPANESE FACIAL MASSAGE

This massage technique originated in Japan and was devised by Mrs Marie Faux-Jones for her colleges in Tokyo and Bath.

More pressure points are used than in a European facial massage. This is both to aid lymphatic drainage and to apply pressure to shiatsu points. Other movements include gliding and circling with the fingertips.

Method
1 Cleanse the face in the usual manner.
2 Apply a light oil to the face.
3 The first movement is an effleurage and contact movement. Pressure is applied behind the ear, then the hands are cupped over the ear. Glide up the face and apply pressure over the bridge of the nose. Smooth over the face and head to apply pressure at the nape of the neck.
4 The diagrams opposite show a sequence of 21 movements. The whole massage takes approximately twenty minutes.

INDIAN EYE CARE

Shahnaz Husain, who has beauty schools in New Delhi and other parts of India, has contributed some simple treatments for the eyes that can be recommended for clients to perform at home. She says that the eyes are probably the most wonderful part of the anatomy; they present us with such a variety of sights. The skin around the eyes is, however, extremely vulnerable. It is thin in texture, and lines and wrinkles very easily. There are no sebaceous glands in this region to produce the oils that keep the skin soft and smooth.

As important as external treatment is, it is also necessary to look at the life style of the client: the kind of food that is eaten, the client's occupation, the amount of sleep that she normally has. The eyes are

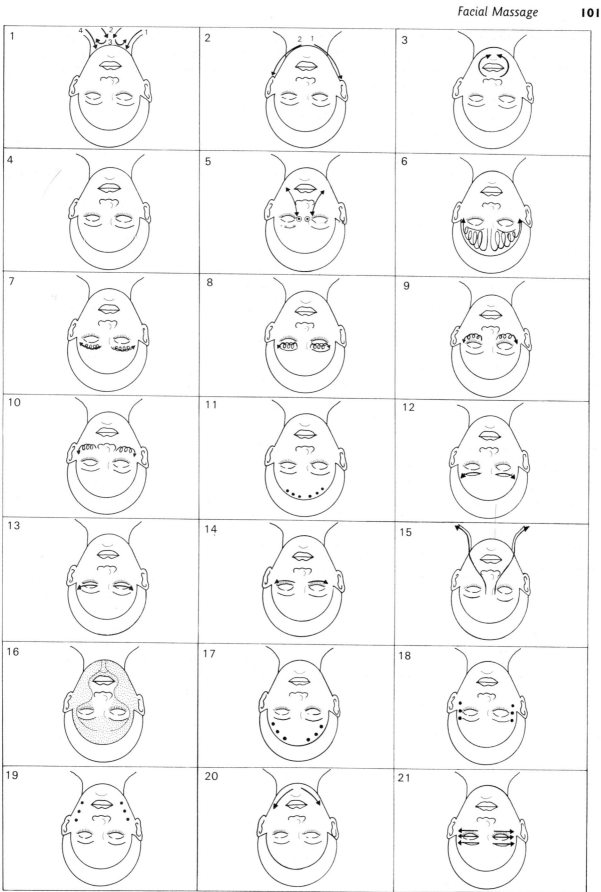

the most overworked features of the face. They can be strained by reading for long periods or by watching too much television. Harsh lights, wind, dust, emotional anxieties, an excess of alcohol and smoking can all be detrimental. The results of so much strain tells on the eye muscles, which become tense and weary, leading to problems of vision and appearance.

Dark Under-eye Circles

This is a common problem which may be caused by lack of sleep, fatigue, stress, dietary deficiency, or disease. In certain conditions, the client may be advised to seek medical assistance. She should be advised to follow a daily beauty routine. Cosmetic products should be chosen with great care, because the skin around the eyes is very delicate. The skin around the eyes should be cleansed every night with a rehydrant gel. An under-eye cream should then be applied. Products that are used around the eyes must be very light in texture. An under-eye cream containing lanolin and almond is ideal. Almond helps to remove dark circles as it is a mild natural bleach. It is also an excellent 'skin food'. Remove the cream after ten minutes. No cream should be left on the skin around the eyes for long periods.

The area around the eyes should be avoided when applying a mask unless it is one specially formulated for this area, such as a seaweed mask in a liquid form. This has a light texture and a watery consistency which forms a light film on the skin, and can easily be removed with water. Seaweed is a moisturiser and also has a revitalising effect on the skin.

Under-eye Bags

This is usually caused by a hereditary problem. They appear like pouches just under the eyes and seem to add years to the face. It is usually during one's thirties that under-eye bags develop and become apparent. Sometimes the pouches may be caused by other reasons, such as sinus problems, urinary tract infections and kidney ailments.

The skin has a tendency to accumulate fluid. Since the skin around the eyes is very thin and delicate, it has very little resilience. When it stretches, it begins to sag.

If there are any internal problems, medical advice should be sought. It is important to keep the kidneys functioning well by drinking adequate quantities of water, as this helps the body to flush out the system. The kidneys help to remove toxins and other waste substances from the body. Advise the client to reduce intake of coffee and tea, and to drink a glass of warm water with the juice of a lemon first thing in the morning. It is said that about one and a half litres of fluid is necessary to keep the kidneys functioning well. A major part of which should be plain water. This will help to keep the eyes looking clear.

Never apply a heavy cream around the eyes or leave any cream on for a long time as this increases puffiness. Potato extract or slices can be applied around the eyes to reduce puffiness. Cucumber juice can also be applied. Stubborn eye-bags that are hereditary may be removed by cosmetic surgery.

Recommend a few eye exercises for the client to perform at home to relieve muscular tension and maintain the health of the eyes.

1 First look at a very close object in front of you and then look at an object as distant as possible. This can be done by facing a window, so that the eyes command a sweeping view.
2 Rotate the eyes in a complete circle without moving the head, first clockwise and then anti-clockwise.
3 With the head erect, move the eyes to first look at the ceiling and then at the floor. Repeat this ten times. Then look to the extreme right and then to the extreme left. Do not squint when the eyes are moved. Between the exercises relax the eyes by closing them tightly and then opening them wide.
4 While performing close work such as reading, shut the eyes for a few seconds from time to time. This will protect them from strain. Even blinking helps the eyes. When blinking occurs, the eyes are bathed by moisture and cleansed. Rest is the best relief for tired eyes.

Chapter 12

Heat and Ultraviolet Treatments

Everyone feels warmth. Most people can see things around them because of light. Most people can hear some form of sound.

All substances are made up of molecules. They are in a constant state of movement. The warmer the molecules are, the faster they move and the matter they make up expands. If the substance is cold, the molecules move more slowly and the matter contracts.

Molecules are made up of a number of atoms. These atoms may all be of the same type, called an *element*. Molecules may be arranged in a set order but made up of more than one atom (a *compound*). The properties of a compound may be different from those of the original elements. A mixture is made up of molecules of more than one type which do not combine to form a new molecule. There are over a hundred known elements. Each is given its own code of letters:

Oxygen   – O
Nitrogen – N
Gold   – Au
Silver   – Ag
Calcium – Ca

The air around the earth is made up of invisible and odourless gases such as oxygen, O; nitrogen, N; and carbon dioxide, CO_2; with traces of other gases including hydrogen. Pure oxygen is written as O. When it is written as O_2 it indicates a balance of two atoms of oxygen in a molecule. Water is shown as H_2O, that is, two atoms of hydrogen and one atom of oxygen in each molecule.

The human body is made up of 29 elements. Ninety per cent of the body is made up of oxygen, hydrogen, carbon and nitrogen. Other elements include calcium, potassium, sodium and iron.

THE ELECTROMAGNETIC SPECTRUM

Heat, light and sound are transmitted through different elements along electromagnetic waves. These waves have *peaks* and *troughs*. The distance between each wave is known as a *wavelength*. In each wavelength the peaks will be the same distance from each other and will travel at the same speed. In some wavelengths, the distance between peaks can be measured in kilometres. Others are so small they are measured in nanometres, shown as 'nm'. These are one ten-millionth of a millimetre. Sometimes the measurement is given in ångström units.

10 ångströms = 1 nanometre.

The number of waves that go through a point at any given time is called a *frequency*. The number of waves per second is measured in *Hertz*.

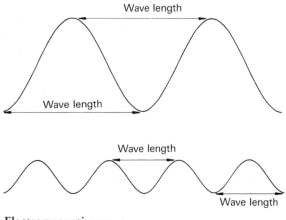

Electromagnetic waves

These waves are arranged in a spectrum from the very short *gamma* waves to the wide *microwaves*. After these come the radio waves. Some of these different groups overlap one another.

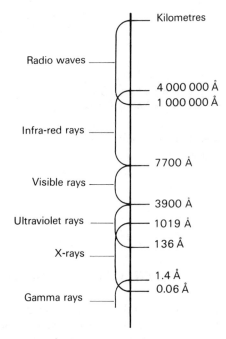

Kilometres

Radio waves

4 000 000 Å
1 000 000 Å

Infra-red rays

7700 Å

Visible rays

3900 Å

Ultraviolet rays

1019 Å

136 Å

X-rays

1.4 Å

0.06 Å

Gamma rays

Electromagnetic spectrum

Everyone knows the colours of a rainbow: violet, indigo, blue, green, yellow, orange, red. These are known as the colours of the *visible light spectrum*. If pure white light is refracted by a prism these colours can be seen in sequence. Visible light rays are only 12 per cent of the output from the sun. The rest are invisible.

The visible rays lie between 3900 Å and 7700 Å in the spectrum. Beyond the violet light are rays that we cannot see. The first are the *ultra* (beyond) violet rays lying between 3900 Å and 136 Å. Ultraviolet rays and the rays beyond them are cold rays, giving off no heat. Ultraviolet light can be classified as UVA, UVB and UVC rays.

UVA Rays

UVA rays lie between 3150 Å and 3900 Å, next to the visible violet rays. They are able to penetrate to the dermis. They have an aesthetic use, in that they tan the skin without burning it. They produce a chemical reaction in the melanocyte cells found in the skin, causing them to produce melanin.

UVB Rays

UVB rays lie between 2800 Å and 3150 Å. These rays are absorbed in the lower layers of the epidermis. UVB rays induce a strong erythema (page 26). They also stimulate the production of *ergosterol* in the skin.

This is required by the body for the production of vitamin D, which aids absorption of calcium and phosphorus (needed for the formation of bone tissue). UVB will cause the skin to thicken and ultimately to burn. The skin may never completely recover from the damage. If the burning is repeated too often, very serious problems can occur, e.g. skin cancer, from the accumulated damage. Both the melanin and the thickening are the body's defence reaction.

UVC Rays

Although given off by the sun, very few UVC rays reach the surface of the earth, as they are absorbed in the outer zones of the earth's atmosphere. UVC rays very quickly produce an erythema and skin cancers often develop. UVC is, however, manufactured for industrial purposes as these rays have a highly germicidal effect.

UVC rays lie below 2800 Å. Below the UVC rays in the spectrum lie the X-rays. The rays with even shorter wavelengths are the gamma rays.

Infra-red Rays

The red rays of the visible light spectrum give off a very small amount of heat. Beyond them lie the longer rays of the invisible infra-red rays which give off significantly more heat. Their wavelengths range from 7700 Å to 4 000 000 Å. Beyond the infra-red rays lie the radio waves and then the ultrasonic waves.

Grotthus–Draper Law

Grotthus–Draper law states that for electro-magnetic waves to have any effect on the body, they must be absorbed in the tissues. The amount of radiation is dependent on a number of variables: the frequency of the rays, the angle at which they strike the skin, the distance from the skin, and the length of time that the skin is subjected to the rays.

The Inverse Square Law

The principle of the inverse square law states that if a light of known power is placed directly over a square that is one square metre, but one metre away from it, a known amount of intensity and light will fall onto that square. One metre beyond this first square lies another square measuring two square metres. It will receive the same amount of light from the original source as the first square. However because it lies two metres away from the light source and is four times the size of the first square the light intensity on it will be a quarter of the amount received by the smaller square.

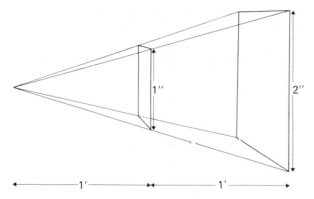

The inverse square law

These are both very important points to remember when positioning any lamp emitting rays over a client.

ULTRAVIOLET

People wanting a cosmetic tan normally use an ultra-violet treatment. Most white-skinned people believe that they look fitter and more attractive if they have a tanned appearance.

UVC penetrates just into the superficial epidermis.
UVB penetrates to the deep epidermal layer.
UVA penetrates into the dermis.

It can take up to 48 hours for any colouration to show up in the skin. Further colouration may occur from 2–19 days after the original exposure. This is one very good reason why ultraviolet treatment should not be given every day.

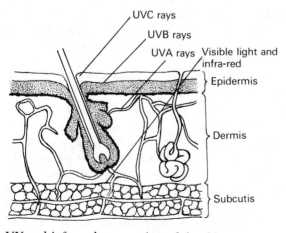

UV and infra-red penetration of the skin

Because it is a powerful source of energy, ultraviolet can cause severe damage to the eyes. As this damage is painless at first, many people are led to believe it is non-existent. Special protective goggles *must* be worn for any ultraviolet treatment. Normal sunglasses are not sufficient. The therapist must also protect her own eyes if working near an ultraviolet unit. The Health and Safety at Work Act states that it is illegal for staff to be working sufficiently near to an untraviolet unit to need eye protection. Ultraviolet rays can be reflected from any light or bright surfaces.

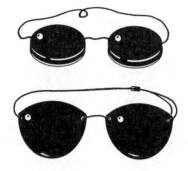

There are several different types of ultraviolet equipment. The older type of solarium has small quartz lamps and possibly infra-red bulbs, or uses lamps similar to the infra-red lamp, which have a filament within them.

Solarium: floor-standing model

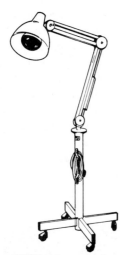

A single-headed treatment lamp

Neither of these types of lamp are now considered suitable for giving an ultraviolet treatment as they both emit UVB.

Some sunbeds are sold as 'high speed' or 'rapid tan' beds. A number of these also emit UVB and should be avoided. There are however, a number of safe sunbeds. Those having a 'high pressure' quartz lamp emit pure UVA.

Ultraviolet equipment must now conform to the British UVA Standard (No. 3456.102.27) which states that there must be a minimum of 99 per cent UVA emission. (See Appendix A, page 199).

Equipment should be installed so that clients cannot touch the radiation lamps. After 600 hours the lamps need to be replaced as their effectiveness will have diminished although there may not be any visible indications. They should be replaced according to the manufacturer's instructions. Any damaged or 'crazed' tubes or bulbs should be replaced immediately.

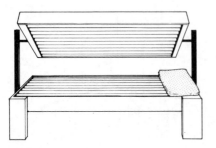

A flat sunbed with canopy

Contra-indications

There are a number of contra-indications to ultra-violet treatment which should be observed. Do not give a suntanning treatment to anyone who:

    does not achieve a tan in natural sunlight
    is ultra sensitive to natural sunlight
    burns easily in natural sunlight
    frequently gets 'cold sores' or has recently had shingles
    suffers from migraine, frequent headaches, epilepsy or who faints easily
    is pregnant
    suffers from certain skin conditions such as eczema or vitiligo
    has had chemotherapy treatment in the previous three months
    suffers from a serious cardio-vascular or lung condition
    has a fever at the time of the proposed treatment
    has received such treatments as electrolysis, skin peeling or depilatory waxing in the past 12 hours
    is on certain forms of medication, e.g. birth control pills or diuretics may cause nausea. Other medicines or tropical preparations can result in severe burning.

If in doubt about a client having a treatment, insist on written permission from their doctor. Further advice may be sought from the Association of Sun Tanning Organisations. (See Useful Addresses, page 204.)

No client should have more than half an hour on each side of the body during a treatment. People who have red hair or sensitive skin should have shorter treatments.

If a client goes into the normal British sun for quarter of an hour they should have half an hour taken off their sunbed time. If the sun is very hot, it is probably better for them not to have the sunbed treatment at all. Sunbed treatments should not be given more often than every other day.

Before every treatment there are a number of things that the therapist should do:

1 Check that the sunbed is in full working order.
2 Make sure that the acrylic surface of the sunbed has been thoroughly cleaned. It is a good idea to wipe it over before each treatment to show the client that a good state of hygiene exists.
3 Place a clean sheet of couch roll on the floor for the client to stand on. This can avoid any risk of passing on such conditions as athletes foot or verrucae.

Before each treatment the client must:

1 Remove all make-up.
2 Shower with a non-perfumed soap.
3 Ensure that the skin is completely dry.
4 Make sure that there is no lotion, perfume, cream, powder, or deodorant on the skin.
5 Remove contact lenses if possible.
6 Cover any hair that has recently been bleached or tinted.
7 *Wear goggles* (see page 105).

During each treatment the therapist should:

1 Stay within call of the client.
2 Check on the client to make sure that they have not fallen asleep or become unwell.
3 Ensure that the client does not receive more than the prescribed exposure to the ultraviolet radiation.

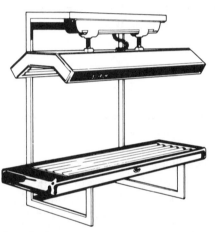

A curved sunbed

After each treatment the client should:

1 Rise from the sunbed slowly, otherwise fainting may occur.
2 Take another shower if necessary, to remove excess sweat.
3 Apply a moisturiser to the face and body to counteract the drying effect of the ultraviolet.

After each treatment the therapist must thoroughly clean the acrylic covering of the sunbed. Great care must be taken not to scratch the acrylic surface otherwise 'light' will not be evenly distributed. Do not use a dry cloth as this can cause static electricity. Use a soft cloth with a mild antiseptic. Do not use surgical spirit or bleach as this can discolour the acrylic.

INFRA-RED

Infra-red rays can be produced by two methods: a *non-luminous* generator or a *luminous* generator.

Non-luminous Generator

This type of generator is rather like an electric fire with the element wrapped around fireclay or even embedded into it. The element emits rays which heat the fireclay. This type of ray is not visible. The infra-red rays are directed onto a curved reflector mounted behind it. The reflector is then positioned so as to reflect the rays where they are required. It is not widely used in the field of beauty because it takes about 10 minutes to become fully heated.

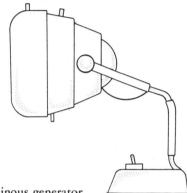

A non-luminous generator

Luminous Generator

This type of generator is like a large electric light bulb. It contains a wire filament which heats in about 30 seconds. When the filament is heated it emits infra-red rays as well as a few rays of visible light. This appears as a warming white light. When intended for use on humans, the bulb is given a red coating.

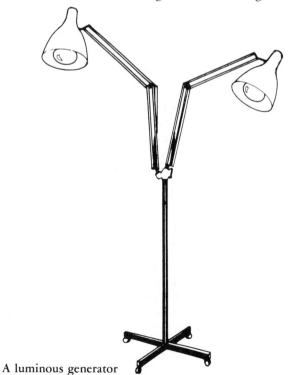

A luminous generator

Infra-red Treatment

Infra-red lamps give off a warming glow reminiscent of the sun. Psychologically this gives people a feeling of well-being and therefore helps them to relax.

Physiologically, infra-red treatments can be given for three main reasons: to produce hyperaemia, to relax tissues or to relieve pain.

Hyperaemia

When tissues are warmed, blood and lymph vessels dilate. The blood flow to that area is increased, bringing nutrients and oxygen. The increase in white blood cells assists in destroying local bacteria, while the removal of waste matter also speeds up. The increased circulation improves the repair of tissues and reduces local congestion. The skin will appear pink and warm after an infra-red treatment.

Relaxing Tissues

Muscles relax when they are warm. This means that many treatments can be more easily performed after an infra-red treatment. Warmth also helps the epithelial skin tissues to relax, thus aiding the introduction of certain substances into the skin.

Relieving Pain

A gentle heat can have a mild sedative effect on sensory nerve endings. A stronger heat can act as a counter-irritation on superficial sensory nerve endings. By relaxing the muscle tissues and speeding up the blood flow, pain caused by recent injury or acute inflammation can be relieved. If too much intense heat is given, it may cause fluid seepage into the tissues and thus actually cause pain.

Treatment for the relief of pain may be given once or twice a day. The time given may be between 20–30 minutes but this time may be exceeded if required. Five minutes is usually considered sufficient time to warm the tissues of the face.

The infra-red rays should be applied directly to the skin. This must be free of oils. Thick pads of cotton-wool should be used to protect the eyes. Contact lenses must be removed prior to a treatment.

The bulb should be positioned at a distance of 45–75 cm (18–30 inches) from the area. The heat should be comfortably warm for the client. If it is too hot, the tissues can be damaged. (See *single-headed treatment lamp*, page 106.)

Following a treatment, care must be taken to see that the area treated does not get cold.

Contra-indications and Precautions

Contact lenses should be removed because they intensify heat and could burn the eyes.

Small areas of sensitive skin or broken capillaries should be protected with thick pads of cotton-wool. On larger areas, protect the skin and position the lamp farther away.

Prolonged infra-red radiation may produce headaches, especially when it is applied to the back for any length of time.

Burning may occur if the lamp is placed too near the skin or the intensity is too great for that person.

Great care should be taken where there is reduced skin sensitivity, as with diabetics.

Do not apply cream or oil to the skin prior to infra-red treatment.

Do not apply to areas where there is a defective arterial blood supply or a danger of haemorrhage.

STEAM

There are several forms of steaming: *hot steam*, *ozone vaporiser*, or *cold steam*.

Contra-indications to Steaming

Sensitive skin (may be protected)

Broken capillaries (may be protected)

Areas of vascular disturbance such as acne rosacea

Areas of broken skin, irritation or abrasion

Skin having a reduced sensitivity, such as diabetes

Hot Steam

This type of equipment produces a heated spray of water. The heater consists of a cylinder containing an element that will heat water to boiling point. The water is projected out of a nozzle which diffuses the steam into a fine mist. This is directed onto the skin, usually the face or back. The purpose of the hot steam is to moisten the skin and warm the underlying tissues.

The client's eyes and any sensitive areas of skin or broken capillaries must be protected by pads of damp cotton-wool. The client's hair, clothing and the couch etc. must also be protected from the steam.

Steam is given for 5–10 minutes, depending on the skin type. The nozzle is positioned 50–75 cm (20–30 inches) away from the skin, depending on the apparatus.

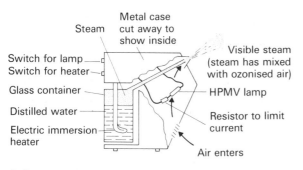

A face steamer

Distilled water should be used in the steamer to reduce 'furring' inside the equipment.

Ozone Vaporiser

Most hot steamers are capable of producing ozone.

The ozone (O_3) is produced by passing steam in front of ultraviolet light; usually a quartz high-pressure lamp. The presence of ozone makes the steam more visible.

Ozone has a highly bactericidal effect. It is therefore useful for local areas of infection or for larger areas of acne. It is not necessary to use it on normally good skin. Ozone should only be used for very short periods of time in a well-ventilated room. The vapour carrying the extra atom of oxygen is believed to have carcinogenic properties.

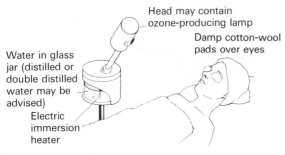

An ozone vaporiser

Cool Steam

The water container should be filled up to the safety mark, preferably with distilled water.

The steam is dispersed along a narrow metal tube. It passes over the end of a plastic tube, the other end of which is placed in a glass container. This may contain a solution such as rose water or skin tonic or just plain water. The solution is drawn up the plastic tube by the steam passing across the top of it. A fine mist of cool steam is then given off. This should be directed over the skin for five minutes.

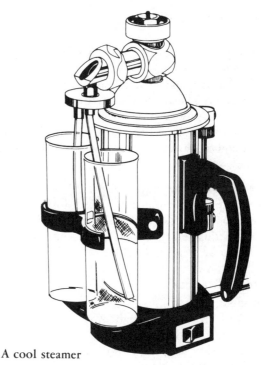

A cool steamer

HEATING PADS

Electrically-heated pads are available in a variety of sizes and shapes.

Some pads are shaped like a cushion and may even have a vibrating unit inside them. Other pads are flat and have a heating element running through them like an electric blanket. When placed on the skin, they warm the superficial tissues.

One unit consists of a face and a neck pads. They can be a little claustrophobic. However, the underlying tissues are pleasantly warmed and relaxed after a treatment of 15–20 minutes.

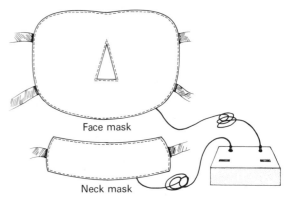

Face pads

Other pads are heated by boiling or by a chemical exchange occurring inside the pad.

PARAFFIN WAX

Paraffin wax is a very pleasant way of warming the tissues and producing an erythema. When heated, paraffin wax is applied to the skin. It gives off its heat quite quickly. The area is therefore usually covered with a plastic sheet and then wrapped in a towel in order to retain heat. The wax usually becomes opaque and cool after 15–20 minutes. It may then be removed.

There are three main ways that paraffin wax can be applied: dipping the area into a wax bath, brushing the wax onto the skin or brushing the wax onto plastic sheeting and then applying the sheeting over the area to be treated.

Contra-indications

Open cuts
Areas of broken skin or abrasion
Any skin condition or irritation
Reduced skin sensation as with diabetes
Areas of defective blood supply, e.g. varicose veins or broken capillaries

Before any paraffin wax treatment, the skin must be clean, dry and free of oil.

Wax Bath

These are 'baths' with a heating element under a container. The wax should be heated to 40–44 °C (104–111 °F). The baths are large enough for a hand or foot to be placed into them. Make sure that the client is not wearing any rings, watches, etc. before placing her hand into the wax bath. The hand or foot is dipped into the wax and then withdrawn so that it forms a wax 'skin'. This is dipped in a further four or five times to build up a good layer of wax. The hand or foot is then placed in a polythene bag and covered with a towel. When it has cooled, remove the towel, polythene bag and wax.

Wax Brushed onto the Skin

A little hot wax is put into a bowl. This is then carefully brushed onto the skin giving it a good covering. The edges of the wax should be straight and firm, as this helps when it is lifted off. When applied to areas of the body other than the face, the wax is covered with a layer of polythene and then wrapped in a towel until it is cool.

When applying wax to the face, the eyes should first be covered with pads of cotton-wool. Hair and clothing must be well protected. Do not apply wax to the eyes, mouth or nostrils. Brush the wax evenly over the skin, building up a layer of 2–3 mm ($\frac{1}{8}$ inch) all over the area. This will form a good mask. It will cool in 5–10 minutes. Remove the wax by gently peeling it off in one piece.

Wax Brushed onto Polythene Sheets

It is sometimes more convenient to apply hot paraffin wax by ladle onto a sheet of polythene. The wax needs to be fairly hot and about 6 mm ($\frac{1}{4}$ inch) thick. The whole sheet is applied to the area of the body to be treated. This is then wrapped in a towel until the wax is cool.

Chapter 13

Electrical Treatments

Before performing any electrical treatment the therapist should have some understanding of the basic physics involved.

SIMPLE PHYSICS OF MOVEMENT

Electricity is a form of energy which, when in motion, causes a thermal or magnetic effect. When it is used in conjunction with other elements it can cause a chemical effect.

Solids, liquids or gases are all different forms of matter. All matter is composed of atoms. These are minute particles which are themselves formed from sub-atomic particles.

The Atom

An atom can be described as having a central nucleus. This is made up of protons and neutrons. Atoms are normally electrically neutral.

Protons

Protons are electrically positive (+) and they carry a positive (+) charge. The number of protons in the atom determines its atomic number. Hydrogen has only one proton so its atomic number is 1.

Neutrons

Neutrons are electrically neutral. Although neutrons carry no electrical charge, their numbers affect the weight of the different atoms and relate to their atomic mass. There are usually the same number of neutrons as protons except in the large elements where the number of neutrons may be greater. Neutrons attach themselves to the protons and prevent them from flying apart.

Isotopes

An isotope is an atom containing the *standard number of protons* for a known element but having a *higher number of neutrons*, thus altering the atomic mass. For example, a carbon atom of the commonest isotope has six protons and six neutrons (carbon-12). Another carbon isotope may have six protons but seven or eight neutrons (carbon-13 or carbon-14).

Electrons

Surrounding the nucleus are the negatively charged (−) electrons. They are usually equal in number to the positively charged (+) protons. They are, however, very much smaller than protons.

Electrons revolve around the nucleus in seven fixed orbits at very high speed. They fill the lowest orbit first. They will not start to fill the next orbit until the previous orbit is full.

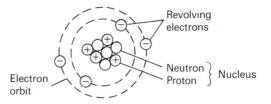

An atom (Beryllium)

The number of electrons in the outer orbit circulating around the nucleus could effect that atom as well as others surrounding it. If there is only one electron rotating in the outer orbit it may join another atom. If a number of electrons rotate in the outer orbit, they are reluctant to enter a chemical combination with other atoms.

A simple atom is of a neutral charge. If it loses an electron, the atom has an excess of positive charge and becomes a positive ion (cation). If it gains an electron the atom then has an excess of the negative charge and becomes a negative ion (anion).

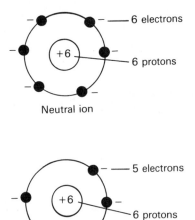

Neutral ion

- 6 electrons
- 6 protons

Positive ion

- 5 electrons
- 6 protons

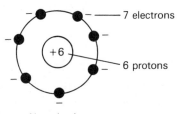

Negative ion

- 7 electrons
- 6 protons

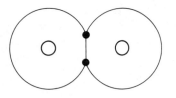

Ions

Combined Atoms

Bonding

When two or more atoms join together they are said to be bonded. They may share two electrons.

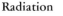

Bonding

Molecules

A molecule is the term for two or more atoms joined together.

Elements

An element is matter made up of only one kind of atom.

Compounds

A compound is matter formed from two or more chemical elements whose atoms are bonded.

Electrovalents

This type of compound occurs because of the attraction of opposites. If one atom gives an electron to the next atom, the first atom becomes a positive (+) ion and the second atom becomes a negative (−) ion.

Covalents

This type of compound occurs when similar atoms share a bonding of electrons.

Mixtures

A mixture is matter made up of atoms of more than one kind. Even when they are mixed together they will not combine.

Radiation

Radiation energy is produced by movement of the electrons within their own atom. If energy or heat is added to an atom, the electrons move outwards to the outer orbit and the atom is said to be in an excited state. When the electron returns to its original orbit it gives off a pulse of electromagnetic energy called a *photon*.

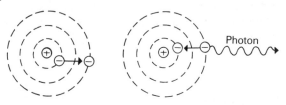

Photon

Radiation

Conductivity

Some atoms have only a few electrons on their outer orbit. This allows the electrons to move to other atoms and so carry a charge of electric current. The electric flow will be in one direction. The elements or compounds containing these atoms are called conductors.

Non-conductors

Atoms which have a number of electrons on the outer orbit are unlikely to lose them because they are held firmly in orbit. They therefore do not conduct an electrical current.

The Power of Attraction

Atoms that are unlike are attracted to each other. For example, negative atoms are attracted towards the positive pole.

Atoms which are alike repel each other, e.g. negative atoms repel other negative atoms.

The greater the number of electrically charged electrons an atom has, the greater its potential for repelling or attracting other electrons.

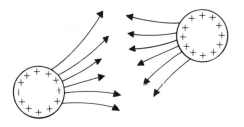

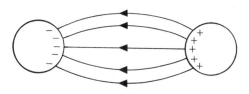

The power of attraction

GALVANISM

Galvanism is a treatment that makes use of the movement of atoms between negative and positive poles. Disencrustation is given to 'pull out' the dirt and iontophoresis to 'push in the goodies'. Much more is understood about the principles involved than a few years ago. There are far more products available now from manufacturing houses worldwide. Chemists have worked out why some materials have a particular effect if used in a certain manner.

Galvanism, when used in beauty therapy, employs the use of a direct electrical current. This is a constant current with no interruption.

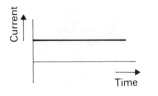

Non-interrupted galvanic current

Frequency less
than 30 Hz

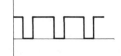

Interrupted galvanic current

The treatment of galvanism is concerned with the movement of ions within the face (or body). If the ions are positive (+) they are called *cations* because they move towards the cathode or the negative electrical pole. If the ions are negative (−) they are called *anions* because they are attracted towards the anode, that is, the positive electrical pole.

Cations and Anions

It must be remembered that:
 like poles repel,
 unlike poles attract.

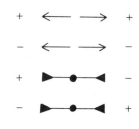

Attraction

Anions

Negative (−) anions produce a strong alkaline reaction on the skin. This is due to sodium hydroxide being produced in the electrolyte. They stimulate the circulation and increase blood and lymph flow to the area, creating a local hyperaemia. They soften keratin and dried sebum and increase the activity of sweat and sebaceous glands. The nerve endings are excited by anions.

Negative (−) anions are attracted to a positive (+) pole and are repelled by a negative (−) pole.

Cations

Positive (+) cations produce an acid reaction on the skin because hydrochloric acid is produced by the electrolyte. This has a more soothing effect. Cations decrease the blood supply to the area and assist in contracting the pores. They have a hydrating effect and will help to restore the acid mantle of the skin.

Positive (+) cations are attracted to the negative (−) pole and are repelled by a positive (+) pole.

The skin has a natural resistance to substances being pushed into it. It is almost impossible to actually push any substance into it. However, ionised substances can be attracted by a good conductivity towards an opposite pole.

It does not matter if the substance being used is a positive (+) cation or a negative (−) anion as long as the correct polarity is being used for the electrode.

Active electrode	Attracts	Propels
Positive	*negative* ions away from the *negative* electrode	*positive* ions towards the *negative* electrode
Negative	*positive* ions away from the *positive* electrode	*negative* ions towards the *positive* electrode

When positive (+) cations are moved the process is called *cataphoresis*.
When negative (−) anions are moved the process is called *anaphoresis*.

Electrodes

There are a number of different electrodes that may be used. For facial treatments, the client holds a plain metal bar which should be wrapped in wet lint. This is usually called the *indifferent*, *neutral* or *passive* electrode. Some people prefer to use a pad electrode strapped to the client's upper arm.

The other electrodes may be called the *direct*, *working* or *active* electrode. These are the ones with which the treatment will be performed. It does not refer to their polarity.

The most commonly used electrode on the face is the roller. Very often the therapist uses one roller in each hand.

Other electrodes come in the shapes of a small ball or pear on the end of a wand, or a pair of forceps. These are useful for working in small crevices such as those found around the nose or under the lower lip. Disc electrodes of varying size may also be used for specific areas.

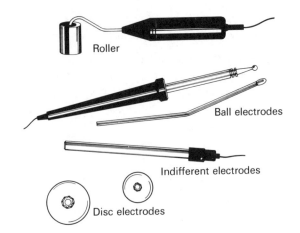

Galvanic electrodes

A mask containing metal plate electrodes may be placed all over the face for a general treatment.

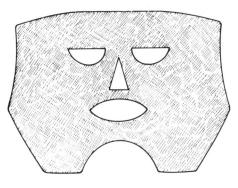

It is important to know what the polarity of both the active and the passive electrodes are, and the ionisation of the solution under them. Knowing the polar and interpolar effects is crucial to performing galvanism effectively. It is far more important to know this than what colour lead is attached to which electrode.

A galvanic machine is usually quite a simple looking one. It will have an on/off switch which may also be used to turn up the amount of current. There is usually an ampere meter which will show the amount of resistance between the two poles. There may be just two outlet apertures labelled '+' or '−', or there may be four or even more outlets. On some machines there may be a switch to change the polarity of the electrodes.

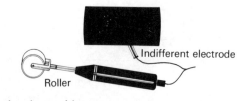

A galvanic machine

The skin must not come into contact with the metal of an electrode at any time while the current is switched on.

It is advisable to wrap the passive electrode in damp lint before handing it to the client. It is a good idea to rest the client's hand on several thicknesses of towelling so that the dampness does not seep through to her. The electrode covering should not be uneven or it will not act as a good conductor.

There are several ways to protect the skin on the face. A heavy, stable gel may be used which does not run off the face. When using a lighter gel or liquid (as from an ampoule) some of the solution should be applied to the skin, and then several thicknesses of wet gauze placed over the face, following its contours. A further layer of gel or liquid should then be applied over the gauze. The rollers may safely be used over this.

All the smaller electrodes should be covered with a layer of good quality cotton-wool firmly held in place with cotton thread or a rubber band. If using the facial mask or pads on the body, all the gel or solution should be applied to the skin and not to the pad. This gives a better contact and the gel is then not wasted. The pads should be fairly wet, not just damp.

Contra-indications

Abrasions, open skin or rashes
Septic areas
Severe broken capillaries
Epilepsy
Diabetes
Clients having a nervous disorder
Clients having any metal pins, plates or pacemakers
Clients having a number of metal fillings may sense an unpleasant metallic taste
Neither the client nor the therapist should wear any jewellery when this treatment is being performed.

Prior to a galvanic treatment, the skin should be gently warmed. On no account should sweating be promoted. The warming may be performed by steaming over gauze, with hot towels or by the use of infra-red heat placed some distance away for just a short time.

The skin must be thoroughly cleansed and all vestiges of oil removed prior to this treatment otherwise there will not be a good conductivity for the ions. By the same token the client's hand holding the passive electrode should also be wiped free of oil.

Amperage

A galvanic treatment may be performed in two ways for two different effects: *iontophoresis* or *desincrustation*.

The ampere meter will give a reading showing the amount of resistance by the skin under the working electrode. Different areas of the face or body will have a different amount of resistance. The output should be adjusted accordingly.

If the amperage is too high, galvanic burning can occur. The amperage should not be more than 0.05 milliamps per square centimetre for the small electrodes and 2.4 milliamps in total for pad-type electrodes.

If two or more working electrodes are used, the output shown will be for the first electrode. The other electrodes will have the same amount of output. If two electrodes are being used the amperage should not be doubled.

When using a negative (−) working electrode the amperage will be low: 0.5–0.6 milliamps (mA) on the ampere meter. It is not necessary to go even this high if the client experiences a sensation.

Even if very low readings are shown on the amperage meter, the treatment will still be working well. The client may feel a slight tingling on the skin. At no time should it feel uncomfortable.

At no time should the skin be allowed to become dry otherwise a galvanic burn can occur.

Iontophoresis

For this treatment a positive (+) substance is most commonly used with a positive (+) working electrode.

Some substances contain both negative (−) and positive (+) ions. In this case the treatment is first performed using the negative (−) working electrode. The output is then reduced to zero. The polarity of the machine is changed, either by a switch or by reversing the plugs at the end of the electrode leads. The treatment is then continued using the working electrode as a positive (+) charge.

Treatment time is usually 4–5 minutes depending on the skin type and sensitivity.

Following iontophoresis using anaphoresis one of three methods may be used to return the skin to its normal acidic state:

1 The polarity of the electrodes can be reversed so that cataphoresis is performed for a short while. This decreases the blood supply to the area, closes the pores and relaxes the skin.

2 The treatment may be followed by high-frequency.
3 A massage can be used to calm the skin.

Iontophoresis using a positive (+) ion (cataphoresis) has a much more gentle effect. It has a hydrating as well as a calming effect. This makes it more useful in cases of acne or hypersensitive skin.

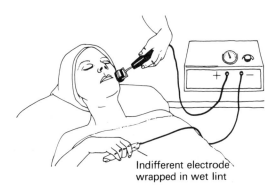

Indifferent electrode wrapped in wet lint

Iontophoresis

Desincrustation

Galvanism can also be used for its cleansing action. It is then normally performed using a negative (−) working electrode. In some instances a positive (+) working electrode and negative (−) solution may be used. The negative (−) working electrode when used with a negative solution softens sebum and dry skin cells, relaxes the pores, stimulates the blood flow to the area, and produces an alkaline reaction on the skin.

The length of time for this part of the treatment is 4–5 minutes for a general cleansing, but it can be used for up to 10 minutes on an oily skin.

Following this cleansing action the polarity of the electrode may be changed so that the working electrode is positive (+) while still using the negative (−) solution. The ions will travel towards the positive pole thereby further loosening dried sebum and cells etc.

The skin should then be cleansed thoroughly using the normal cleansing method to remove the impurities dislodged by this treatment. The treatment may then be followed by iontophoresis, high frequency or massage as required. Make-up should not be applied for several hours following a treatment.

After use the electrodes should be thoroughly cleaned and sterilised.

FARADISM

This is a form of passive exercise. The muscles are made to contract by passing an electrical current through them. This current is accepted by the body and has no harmful effects if the treatment is carried out correctly.

Passive exercise means that a muscle, or set of muscles, can be moved (shortened) without the conscious effort of the client.

Faradism will do nothing to reduce fat, but by toning the muscles will give the appearance of a slimmer body. When applied on the face it tightens up sagging muscles, giving a more youthful appearance.

A faradic current generally has a frequency of 50–100 Hz (hertz). Very occasionally this may be 25–125 Hz. It is deemed to be a short-duration, interrupted direct current having a pulse duration of 0.1–1 milliseconds. The current usually has an interrupted surge which produces a muscle contraction. This is then followed by a rest period.

There are four types of surge pattern:
a) *Saw-toothed* There is a gradual build-up of the current and a sudden release of the contraction.
b) *Triangular* There is a gradual build-up of the current followed by a gradual release.
c) *Trapezoidal* There is a gradual build-up of current which is maintained for a short period and then gradually released.
d) *Rectangular* There is a sudden surge of current which is maintained for a short time and then a sudden release of the contraction.

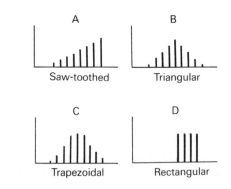

Surge patterns

In some instances the pauses between the surges will follow a regular pattern. In others, there will be an irregular length of time so that the muscles do not 'know' when to expect the next contraction. These patterns can be further altered by having a variation in the length of each surge.

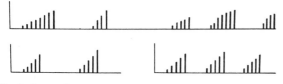

Variations of surge pattern

The reason for having these variations is that the nerve supplying the muscles becomes accustomed to a regular pattern of contraction. This is known as *accommodation*.

The tissues of the body are able to conduct electricity because the tissue fluids contain ions. Muscles have a good supply of blood and are therefore a good conductor. Fatty tissue has little moisture and is therefore a poor electrical conductor. The epidermis layer of the skin also contains very little moisture. When a faradic current is applied to the skin a prickling sensation is felt as the sensory nerve endings are stimulated. This will cause a vasodilation of the superficial blood vessels producing a localised erythema.

The Effects of Faradism

These include:

1 improvement of muscle tone, either in specific groups or in individual muscles
2 shortening of over-stretched muscles
3 increased metabolism so that the tissues require extra oxygen and nutrients
4 increased blood flow to the area causing hyperaemia
5 increased blood and lymph flow away from the area so that toxins and waste matter are removed
6 stimulation of nerve endings so that the nerve pathway is excited
7 re-education of muscles following a prolonged period of inactivity.

Contra-indications to Facial Faradism

General skin diseases or disorders
Local infection or irritations
Local cuts, abrasions or scar tissue
Local bruising
Circulatory conditions: local dilated capillaries, pacemakers, thrombosis, haemophilia, high blood pressure
Neurological disorders: epilepsy, Bell's palsy, neuralgia, neuritis
Localised sensitivity
Highly-strung or nervous people
Migraine sufferers

Faradic type current may be applied to the face in two main ways: *individually*, or in *muscle groups*.

The skin should be thoroughly cleansed before the electrodes are attached so as to allow for the best possible conductivity. The skin should also be warmed so that the tissues are relaxed.

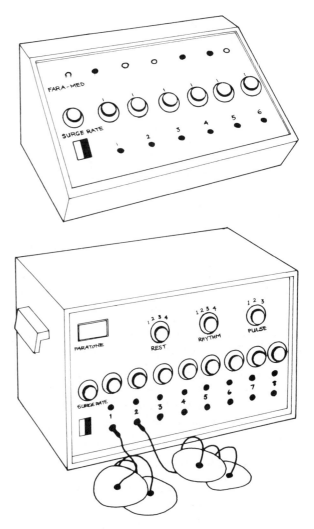

A faradic machine

Individual Muscle Stimulation

In this form of faradism each muscle is stimulated independently of the surrounding muscles. The muscles are activated by stimulation of the motor points (page 50).

The indifferent or passive electrode should be firmly secured to the client so that it cannot become dislodged. This may be under the shoulder, on an arm or even on the upper pectoral muscle. For a good conductivity it should be dampened with a saline solution or wiped with a mild antiseptic. The active (or working) electrode is a small disc. This should be covered in lint or heavy gauze, soaked in a mild antiseptic solution, saline or even plain water.

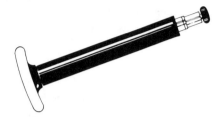

Disc electrode

The active electrode is placed on the motor point of the muscle to be treated. Great care must be taken to trace the motor point. The more accurate the 'pointing' the more easily the electrical current will flow. If the 'pointing' is not accurate the client may suffer a greater degree of prickling discomfort and increased erythema.

A low surge rate of 35–40 per minute should be chosen. The intensity should be raised until a good contraction is seen. It should not be uncomfortable. Because muscle fatigue will occur quite quickly on the smaller facial muscles, the duration should not be longer than 2–3 minutes on each muscle.

After the individual muscle has been exercised, the procedure is repeated on the next muscle.

This is a rather lengthy and time-consuming method of performing this treatment. It is therefore not often used as a general faradic facial treatment but only for specific conditions.

Group Muscle Stimulation

There are several methods of performing this form of faradic facial treatment:

1 roller
2 mask
3 twin electrode.

Roller Method

This consists of a roller which is covered with doeskin or heavy lint (page 114). This is always used wet, having been soaked in weak antiseptic, saline solution or even plain water. The indifferent or passive electrode is usually a pad containing graphite. This pad is firmly secured to the client.

The surge rate should be set at 35–40 per minute. The electrical intensity is set at zero. The damp roller is placed on the skin and must not be removed until

the treatment is completed. A slow, continuous rolling movement should be used throughout. The intensity should be increased until a good muscle contraction is seen.

The treatment should start with two minutes on each side of the face. This is increased by one minute each side until a total of fifteen minutes each side is reached. The benefits are not usually seen until the fifth or sixth treatment. A course of ten treatments should be recommended for the client. Treatments should be three times a week.

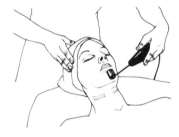

Roller treatment

Mask Method

This method is often used because it incorporates an interferential current. A medium-frequency current is placed in two diagonal positions to produce a low-frequency effect where the currents cross. The electrodes may be in the form of dampened pads or strapping.

The two frequencies need not be of the same hertz value. In fact the frequency can be altered so as to produce a variable effect. If pads are used, they may be moved around the outside of the face to vary the position of the low-frequency intensity.

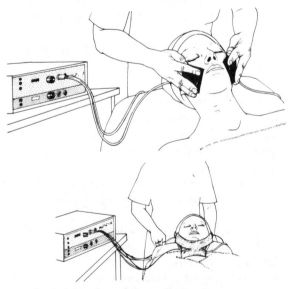

Interferential pads and strapping

One of the problems of using a fixed padding is that the area of greatest intensity lies in the centre of the face. If pads are used, the therapist's hands can be moved to find the area where this treatment is required.

The intensity is turned up until a good contraction is seen. The treatment will last 5–15 minutes.

Twin Electrode Method

This type of electrode has both the indirect (passive) electrode and the active electrode built into it.

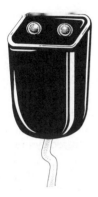

Twin electrode

The method of treatment is similar to the individual muscle stimulation. The electrode is placed on one muscle at a time, although there is some electrical seepage into the surrounding tissues. This is because the electrode is unable to pinpoint the motor point very accurately. Some people move the electrode over the skin in a regular rhythm, rather like using the roller to exercise the muscles in groups.

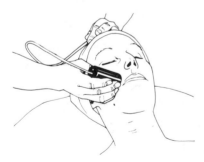

Using a twin electrode

Because faradism can be quite uncomfortable when used on the face, great care must be used to allay any fears that the client may feel. One way to relax the client after this treatment is to perform some soothing facial massage movements. The client could also be shown how to perform certain facial exercises for use between her visits on alternate days.

After each treatment the electrode must be wiped with disinfectant or sterilised, either with a bactericide or by placing in a vapour steriliser.

VACUUM SUCTION

A vacuum suction treatment may be used to break down toxins, fatty tissue and waste matter, and to stimulate the venous and lymphatic systems into removing waste products from the area. Vacuum suction will not remove waste products. Only the body itself can do this.

Vacuum suction can also be used for stimulating tissues (such as the vascular system by producing an erythema), stimulating sensory nerve endings, light muscle toning and the evacuation of comedones.

Vacuum suction works on the principle of a negative pressure, that is, air is drawn out of the cup thus creating a vacuum. When used on the face the negative pressure depends very much upon the condition and flaccidity of the skin. The equipment may be fitted with a gauge to show the amount of vacuum that is produced when the cup is sealed to the skin. The gauge may be calibrated in terms of the length of a column or mercury or as a percentage of atmosphere. In this case the percentage of mercury may be used at 5–10 per cent for lymphatic drainage and 15 per cent for comedone removal. Not more than one third of the cup should be filled by the lifting of the tissue.

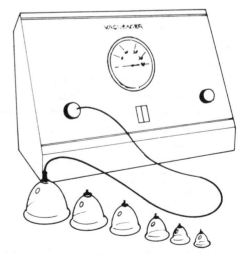

Vacuum suction machine

The equipment consists of a pump (powered by an electrical motor) attached to one of a series of cups by a tube.

There are two different types of cup:
non-breakable plastic, known as *Plexiglass*
shaped glass.

Plexiglass

These cups are simple, round-lipped cups. They are
made in a clear, toughened material and come in four
or five sizes. They are easily cleaned and sterilised in a
liquid steriliser. Do not place them in an autoclave or
an ultraviolet steriliser as this could damage them. If
a cup becomes chipped or crazed it should be
discarded as this could cut the client. It could also
alter the pressure inside it.

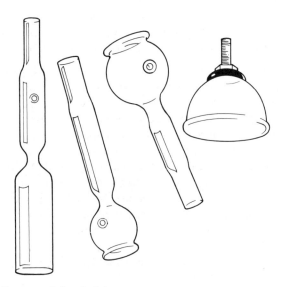

Cups used for facial vacuum suction

Glass Cups

These cups are very fragile. They usually contain a
single hole for the purpose of holding or releasing
the air contained within them. They are made in
different shapes and sizes: they may be round, flat or
have a small aperture for comedone removal. Some
glass cups are also used for work on the body. They
are much more difficult to clean than the simple
Plexiglass cups. A plug of cotton-wool or gauze can
be inserted into them occasionally to absorb any oil
or debris. They should be cleaned and sterilised each
time after use.

The plastic tubing should be thoroughly cleaned each
time it is used. This may be done by soaking in a hot
solution of detergent and then running clean water
through it to remove any oil or debris. It should then
be soaked in a disinfectant and allowed to dry before
re-use.

Contra-indications

Vacuum suction on the face should not be used over:
broken capillaries
fine or sensitive skin
loose or mature sagging skin
delicate skin around the eyes
infected areas
recent scar tissue.

There are two methods of performing vacuum
suction: *gliding* and *tapotement*. Prior to all vacuum
suction treatments the skin should be cleansed and
warm.

Gliding Method

1 Apply a light oil to the area to be treated.
2 Use either a small Plexiglass cup or a small round
   glass cup.
3 Place the cup on the skin to exclude the air.
4 Lift the cup slightly, and take in a gliding movement to the appointed lymph node.
5 Break the suction in a *Plexiglass* cup by inserting
   the little finger of the hand holding the cup, under
   the edge of the cup. The tissue is then depressed
   thus breaking the vacuum. If using a *glass* cup,
   release the finger held over the hole so that air
   enters the cup. The cup should never be pulled off
   the skin. This causes bruising and broken capillaries.

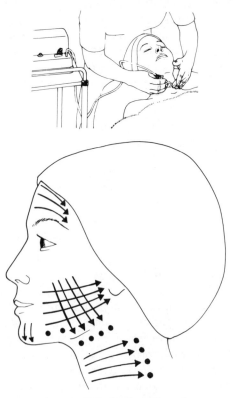

Vacuum suction on the cheek and neck

The first treatment should last 3–5 minutes. This should be increased by two minutes a treatment until a maximum of 10–15 minutes is reached. A course should consist of ten treatments, preferably three times a week. Not much improvement will be seen until the fifth or sixth treatment has been completed.

hyperaemic to occur as well as the breaking down of local waste matter. It is particularly beneficial when used over lines on the forehead. The flat cup is also useful over frown lines in this area.

Comedones may be removed using the glass cup with a small, round aperture. This is used over a dry skin without oil.

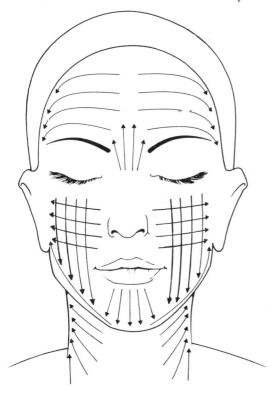

General facial vacuum suction

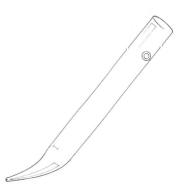

Comedone extractor

The aperture is placed over the comedone and suction increased by positioning a finger over the air hole. The comedone may then be extracted and the vacuum is then released. This form of vacuum suction is not always satisfactory.

Tapotement Method

For this form of vacuum suction treatment the glass cups with an air hole are used. A tapotement or pulse effect may be obtained by lifting and replacing the finger in fairly rapid succession over the air hole. This causes a variation in the negative pressure within the cup.

The cup may be kept static in one area or may follow a glide pattern. The tapotement causes a rapid

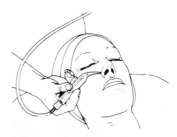

Vacuum suction on the nose

Vacuum suction must be very carefully performed at all times, otherwise the client may feel discomfort and skin and capillaries can be damaged.

When used correctly, vacuum suction may be used to improve several conditions. The blood flow is increased, bringing oxygen and nourishment to the area. Fatty deposits and waste matter can be broken down. The venous and lymphatic flow is stimulated to remove waste products. Lines and wrinkles may be smoothed, and comedones and debris may be expressed.

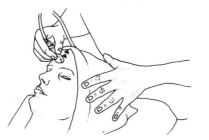

Vacuum suction on the forehead

HIGH-FREQUENCY

A high-frequency current is an electrical current that oscillates at a high speed. It is passed through an electrode, usually made of glass. This contains an inert gas, usually argon or neon, which gives off a blue or pinkish light within the electrode.

The noise is caused by the variation of frequency produced during the treatment by the electronic circuitry. The noise can sometimes be disturbing to a client, who must be reassured before the treatment can commence.

Electrodes are available in a number of different shapes and sizes depending on the purpose for which they are to be used.

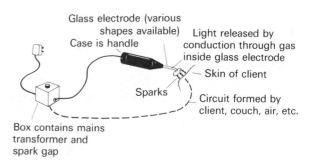

High-frequency circuit

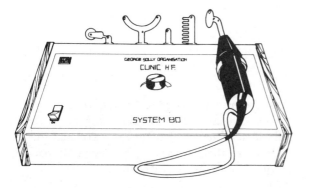

Clinical high-frequency model

One of the most frequently used is the *surface electrode* shaped like a mushroom. It is available in several sizes and is the easiest to use on the face and neck.

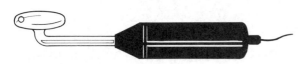

Mushroom-shaped electrode

The *curved electrode* is useful for the neck or for stroking up the arms. The *roller electrode* is rolled back and forth over a larger area such as the back. A *rake* or *comb electrode* is used on the scalp and hair. A *cup-shaped electrode* is used for warming and stimulating the breasts. The *saturator electrode* is normally made of glass and may contain a metal coil inside it; it is held by the client during indirect treatment. There are many other forms of electrodes, but they are used for specific treatments or medical purposes.

High-frequency treatment creates a localised warmth which has a relaxing effect on the tissues. It stimulates the subcutaneous tissue, and particularly the blood circulation, so that nutrients are brought to the area and waste matter is removed. High-frequency also stimulates the sensory nerve endings. Sparking produced by discharge causes atmospheric oxygen to break down and produce ozone. This tends to have a drying effect on the skin as well as acting as an anti-bacterial agent.

High-frequency may be used in two main ways: *direct* and *indirect*.

Direct High-frequency

This form of high-frequency treatment may be used in three different ways:

> fulguration
> gliding
> sparking.

Before any high-frequency treatment is performed, both the client and the therapist must remove all metal jewellery. Failure to do so could result in sparking taking place where there is contact with metal. If it is impossible to remove a piece of jewellery such as a bangle, the skin near it should be protected by tissues.

Neither the client nor the therapist should be in contact with any metal such as a trolley, couch, stool etc.

The therapist should not touch the client (except when performing indirect high-frequency), her clothing or covering or even the couch during the treatment.

Contra-indications

Any area of abrasion, rash or recent scar tissue.
Areas of oedema or blocked sinuses.
Clients who suffer from headaches, migraine or high blood pressure.
Clients who have heart conditions or who wear pacemakers.
Clients who suffer from epilepsy or asthma.
Clients who are pregnant.
Facial treatments should not be given where clients have an excessive number of metallic teeth fillings.

The skin should be thoroughly cleansed before any high-frequency treatment is performed.

Fulguration

A special glass electrode is used to cauterize warts or skin tags. High-frequency may also be used to bleach brown ageing spots found on the back of the hands.

This method should only be used by people fully trained and qualified to use it.

Gliding

In this method an electrode is used to glide over the surface of the skin. Usually a light oil is applied to the area to be treated. In some instances pure talc may be used.

Method

1 Place the electrode on the client's forehead. The client should be warned what to expect.
2 Switch on the high-frequency machine and raise the current to a suitable level.

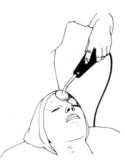

Commencing direct high-frequency

3 Remove your hand from the machine. (At no time should the therapist touch any part of the client or her clothing or any material covering her.)
4 Keep your hand firmly in control of the electrode handle, holding it at the broad, round tube, not at the cone-shaped end.

5 Move the electrode in even lines or in a circular movement in a flat plane to the skin. The electrode should not be lifted up from the skin or sparking will occur. If the electrode is held at an angle to the skin there is a concentration of high-frequency current where it touches the skin. This can cause over-stimulation or even a burn.

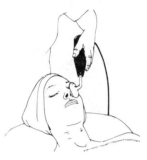

Working around the nose

Great care must be taken when working around the nose. The electrode should be kept as flat as possible. At no time should the electrode be kept in one position for longer than a few seconds, otherwise skin damage can occur.

6 At the completion of the treatment the electrode should be gently moved in a circular fashion. Slowly turn down the high-frequency current and then switch it off before removing the electrode from the skin.
7 Remove the oil from the skin.

The treatment time for the whole face should not normally exceed 8–10 minutes.

Sparking

This can be performed in two different ways: *tapotement* or *over gauze*.

TAPOTEMENT

In this method the electrode is lifted and used in a rapid tapping movement. High-frequency should not be used for longer than five seconds continuously over one area. The electrode should never be lifted further than 5 mm ($\frac{1}{4}$ inch) from the skin. A layer of ozone will be created under the electrode. This will have a drying and anti-bacterial effect. This method is easily employed during a gliding treatment where an area of over-active sebaceous glands require attention.

OVER GAUZE

If the whole face area requires a general stimulation then this method is best employed.

The face is covered in several thicknesses of damp gauze. The electrode is used in the same manner as for the gliding technique. Great care must be taken when going near the eyes, around the mouth or over the nose. Do not touch the gauze whilst using the high-frequency.

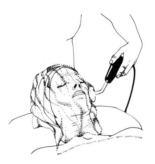

Sparking over gauze

Indirect High-frequency (Viennese Massage)

This is a much more gentle way of using high-frequency. It may be used on dry, mature or sensitive skin to stimulate the underlying tissues. Dry or lifeless skin will be improved, because of the gentle increase in the stimulation of the various body systems.

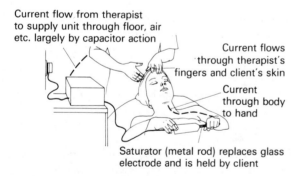

Current flow from therapist to supply unit through floor, air etc. largely by capacitor action

Current flows through therapist's fingers and client's skin

Current through body to hand

Saturator (metal rod) replaces glass electrode and is held by client

Indirect high-frequency circuit

The client's face is cleansed in the usual manner prior to a high-frequency treatment.

Method

1 Give the client the indifferent electrode to hold in one of her hands. It is a good idea to lay a folded towel across her body (under the electrode and holder) in case any sparking should inadvertently take place.

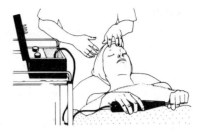

Commencing indirect high-frequency

2 Place one of your hands upon the client's forehead.
3 With your free hand, switch on the machine and raise the high-frequency current to an acceptable level.
4 Place your free hand on to the client's face.
5 Using both hands, perform various facial massage movements. Care should be taken to see that at least part of each hand remains in contact with the client, otherwise sparking will occur, much to the discomfort of the client. A *soothing* form of massage may be performed using effleurage-type movements for a relaxing massage. A *stimulating* massage may be performed using both soothing and tapotement movements. Again, a part of each of your hands must remain in contact with the client. Care should be taken not to work too near to the clients eyes or mouth.
6 The advised time for such a treatment is 10–15 minutes.
7 At the end of the massage, revert to soothing movements, remove one hand and reduce the high-frequency current. Switch off the machine, then remove your second hand.

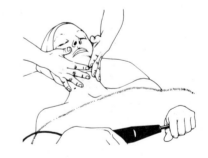

Indirect high-frequency

FACE-LIFTS

There comes a time in every woman's life when she catches sight of herself in a mirror and realises that the years have caught up with her. Her skin has become wrinkled. Her jowl has become heavier.

What can be done to help this woman? The obvious answer is plastic surgery. However, any surgery can be dangerous and should not be undertaken lightly.

There are several things that the therapist can do to help. A regular facial massage is the best way to keep the skin soft and supple and can help to keep the wrinkles at bay. Exercising the facial muscles will help them to keep in tone.

The therapist can perform a 'non-surgical face-lift'. This treatment can be performed on a person of any age. The results will vary depending on the client's age and the condition of the skin and underlying tissues. For a client aged 30 years, a course of ten treatments should be sufficient. The result may last as long as six months. For a client aged 60 years, about twenty treatments would be required, and the result would probably last for only about four months.

Contra-indications

The contra-indications are the same as for normal vacuum suction, faradism and high-frequency.

Method

1 Cleanse, tone and warm the skin in the usual way.
2 Apply a light massage oil to the skin.
3 Use a small, glass vacuum suction cup to perform tapotement all over the area.
4 Change to a small, round Plexiglass cup and continue with the gliding method in the advised manner.
5 The first treatment should last 4 minutes. Increase this by 2 minutes a treatment up to 12 minutes over the course of treatments.
6 To treat the cheeks, glide down to the submandibular lymph nodes below the angle of the jaw. Also glide across the cheeks to the anterior auricular lymph nodes.
7 To treat a small double chin, move the cup up to the cervical lymph nodes. On a large double chin, move the cup down to the clavicular lymph nodes and then to the axillary lymph nodes.
8 Cleanse the skin of all the oil with a mild spirit solution or a strong skin tonic.
9 Now use the faradic current. Dampen the flat electrode and attach it securely.
10 Apply the active electrode. Raise the current until there is a good movement of the muscles. Keep the surge rate low.
11 Commence the treatment with 2 minutes to each side of the face. Increase the time by 2 minutes a treatment up to a total of 10 minutes.
12 Apply a light oil to the face and stimulate the tissues with direct high-frequency. A good blend of neroli, jasmine or other aromatherapy oils may be used instead of plain oil.
13 Complete the treatment with a good, relaxing facial massage.
14 Apply a light mask and then moisturiser.

Treatments should be performed at least three times a week; more if possible in the first week to be really effective.

BREAST TREATMENTS

Breasts are primarily made up of fat, lymph glands and vessels, and lactic ducts, all held in place by the pectoral muscles. The size of the breasts is influenced by hormone activity. Thyroid gland activity can lead to the breasts being too small or over-large. The ovaries also play a part in their appearance, while the pituitary gland produces prolactin which will encourage lactation. When a woman starts to slim she will invariably find that her breasts decrease in size.

Some women feel that they are 'over-endowed' in this part of their anatomy. Others feel that nature has been less than generous here. This is the one attribute that women are particularly sensitive about. They often, therefore, consult the therapist about changing the shape of their breasts.

There are several things that a woman can do for herself, such as exercise. Water treatment apparatus is also available. This is rather a time-wasting form of treatment if performed in a salon perhaps twice a week only. It can have a good tonic effect if used twice a day at home, preferably using a mixer tap, alternating warm and cold water. The client should be shown how to perform bust strengthening exercises.

A wide variety of treatments can be performed at the same time in order to tone up the breasts.

Breast Toning

Vacuum suction is considered to be a useful treatment for reducing slightly over-large breasts. It enables fat to be taken into the axillary lymph nodes, providing the client is on some form of reducing diet. A little extra fat can sometimes be added to the breasts using this same method though this can be a lengthy process.

Faradism is used to exercise the muscles and restore muscle tone.

Contra-indications

These are the same as for normal vacuum suction, faradism and high-frequency.

Method

1 Switch on the machine, with the surge rate at 40–50 per minute, depending on the physical condition of the client.
2 Apply dampened pad electrodes and hold these securely in place.
3 Switch on the current for the first set of pads and turn it up, to a point where contractions are visible.
4 Repeat this for the other sets of pads.
5 Turn up the current on all the pads to show a good overall contraction.

The initial treatment should last 15 minutes; increase this to 25 minutes during the course of ten treatments.

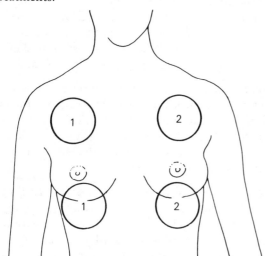

Faradic padding

Bust-lift

Method

1 Warm the area with radiant heat.
2 Stimulate the area with a light hand-held vibrating machine or by manual tapotement.
3 Apply vacuum suction to reduce or augment the fat. A smallish cup only should be used on the area under the nipple. Commence with a low pressure of 6–7 pounds, depending on the age and condition of the client. Increase by one pound at each treatment, until a maximum of 10–12 pounds is reached.
   The initial treatment should last 15 minutes, with treatment time rising to 25 minutes over the course.
4 Remove all the oil with skin tonic, as it will act as an inhibitor to faradism.
5 Apply the faradic pads to the pectoral muscles.

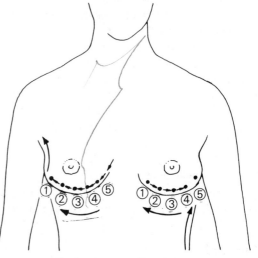

Bust reduce   Bust increase

6 Turn up the current until the muscles are contracting comfortably. The first treatment should last 10 minutes, increasing to 25 minutes by the last session.
7 Apply a light massage oil. A stimulating aromatherapy oil such as lemongrass may be used if preferred.
8 Warm and stimulate the tissues with high-frequency. Use the mushroom-shaped electrode or the special bell-shaped electrode. If using the *mushroom*: gently work around the breasts in a circular movement. If using the *bell*: place the electrode over the nipple. Release the air from the electrode with the pump to create a vacuum. Turn the machine to a low intensity and hold this position for 5 minutes. Repeat on the other breast.
9 Complete the treatment with soothing effleurage-type movements.
10 Remove any surplus oil.

This complex treatment should be carried out three times a week for a course of at least ten treatments.

Chapter 14

Manicure and Pedicare

MANICURE

The purpose of a manicure is to keep the hands and nails in good condition.

A manicure lifts the nail wall and cuticle from the nail plate, so reducing the risk of hangnails. Fragile nails can be strengthened. A hand massage increases the suppleness and flexibility of the hand and wrist, and increases the blood circulation, thereby improving the texture of the skin. With the correct shaping of the nail, the shape of the whole hand can be enhanced. (For anatomy details see Chapter 9.)

A good manicure should help the client to both look and feel better.

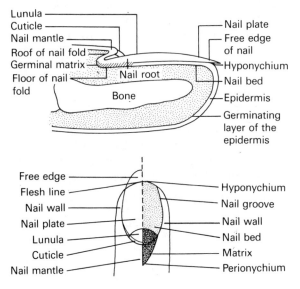

DISORDERS AND CONDITIONS AFFECTING THE NAILS

Age

Although not a disorder, age can affect the nails. The blood supply may be decreased so that there is a lack of such nutrients as iron and calcium. The nails may become thickened, especially the toenails. They may become more opaque. Longitudinal ridges may become more pronounced and numerous. They may split more easily because of a lack of moisture.

Beau's Lines

This is a single transverse furrow affecting all the nails. It is usually caused by an illness such as a severe case of measles, or a thrombosis, when the nails are starved of nutrients. When the physical condition improves, so does the poor condition of the nail.

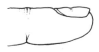

Brittle Nails

This is caused by a poor blood supply to the matrix, resulting in a low fluid content in the nail. It may also be caused by the use of over-strong detergents or solvents which remove the natural oils from the nails. Anaemia or iron deficiency can cause the nail plate to become thinner. Sometimes the nails are so fragile that the free edge curves over the end of the finger.

Cuticle cream should be massaged over the nail plate and matrix each night to increase the blood supply and replace moisture in the nail.

Bruised Nails

When a nail receives a heavy blow, a bruise or blood spot may show through as a dark patch. It will grow out with the nail. If the blow was a very severe one the nail may become detached from the nail base. A new nail will grow normally to replace it.

Chilblains

These usually occur only in the cold weather. They are caused by poor circulation. Swellings occur at the ends of the fingers and toes, around the joints and around the nails. They can be very painful. A manicure or pedicare should not be given over the affected area. Hands and feet should be kept warm and exercise and massage given to improve the circulation once the condition improves.

Dermatitis and Eczema

These two conditions may be hereditary but are more likely to be caused by an irritant. These may include caustic alkalis sometimes found in strong washing powders. They are also sometimes found in cuticle remover. Substances causing problems could include *lanolin* found in some hand and cuticle creams, *resins* found in nail hardeners and nail polishes, and some ingredients used in nail extensions.

Hangnails

This is a sharp spike of nail that has become separated from the side of the nail plate. It may be caused by the nail being excessively dry, rough handling of the cuticle or injury to the matrix.

Hang nail

Hypertrophy

Hypertrophy of the nail may be due to increasing age, damage to the nail bed or general physical disorders such as tuberculosis. The nails may become thickened and misshapen.

Onychauxis (Claw Nail)

This is an excessive thickening of the nail, usually as a result of damage to the matrix or nail bed. In some instances it may resemble a claw. The nail may be made thinner by filing across the top of it and then shaping it as usual.

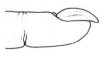

Ingrowing Nail

This occurs mostly in toenails. It is caused by shaping the nail too low at the sides so that they grow into the nail wall.

Koilonychia (Spoon-shaped Nails)

In this condition the nails are splayed, having a depression in the middle and rising to the edges like a spoon. They are often caused by iron anaemia.

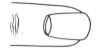

Lamellar Dystrophy (Flaking Nails)

This condition may be due to a poor diet, lacking in vitamins A and B_2. The frequent use of detergents or general poor health may also cause them. The nails tend to break easily. They split across, or even below the free edge in strips. These nails need to be kept short. Good general care is required.

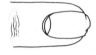

Leuconychia (White Spot)

White spots are caused by air bubbles lying within the layers of the nail. These may be due to damage to the matrix or nail plate. They will grow out with the nail.

Longitudinal Ridges

These tend to occur more frequently in middle-aged people. They may be caused by damage to the matrix or by poor circulation resulting in a calcium or iron deficiency. Buffing with a chamois leather may stimulate the blood flow as well as reducing the ridges.

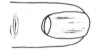

Oncholysis (Separating of Free Edge)

The nail is separated prematurely at the free edge or from the nail wall. It may be caused by using a sharp instrument under the free edge, by the application of false nails or nail extensions, by dermatitis or a fungal infection. Frequent use of an antiseptic may prevent bacteria entering the space under the nail plate. Care should be taken to see that it is not accidentally lifted and broken further.

Pitting

Small pits develop all over the nails. It may be caused by dermatitis, psoriasis or alopecia areata. The nails may become very weak and usually require medical attention.

Psoriasis

Silver scales may develop all around as well as under the nails. The nail may become horny and discoloured. Pitting may occur. Medical attention is required.

Ringworm

This is caused by a fungus (tinea). It appears as a yellowish-brown colour at the free edge, and spreads from the nail bed to the nale plate and then all around the nail. The nail may become thickened. Medical advice should be sought. It is highly contagious.

Splitting Nails

Nails may split when they are thin and brittle and especially where there are ridges. They may also split as a result of poor filing and a general lack of care.

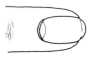

Tinea Pedis

This is commonly called *athletes foot*, and is another form of ringworm. The skin between and under the toes becomes swollen, white and waterlogged. It is highly contagious.

Warts

These may appear on the hands, particularly where there are hangnails. They are caused by a virus. They appear as raised, discoloured patches. They may be rough or smooth. On the feet they may become plantar warts or veruccae, embedded into the skin. All warts are contagious.

Whitlow

This is an acute bacterial inflammation occurring around the nail. The area becomes swollen and painful and is accompanied by pus. Medical attention may be necessary.

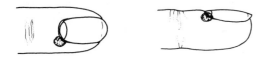

Contra-indications to a Manicure or Pedicare

Any inflammation or infection of the nail, nail wall or cuticle, whitlows, fungal infection, warts, veruccae, severely bruised nails, recent scar tissue, cuts or abrasions close to a nail or an allergy to products.

Instruments and Materials for a Manicure

Instruments

Long emery boards
Orange sticks
Spatulae
Nail brush
Small nail brush
Hoof stick
Cuticle clippers
Manicure scissors
Buffer
Manicure bowl
Small bowl for water
Small bowl for client's jewellery
Receiver for waste material
Towels
Cushion

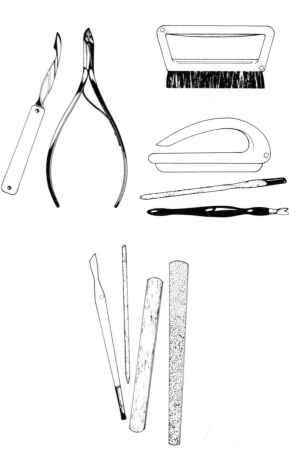

Materials

- Cotton-wool
- Tissues
- Liquid soap
- Antiseptic solution
- Nail polish remover
- Cuticle massage cream
- Cuticle remover
- Hand cream
- Buffing paste
- Pumice stone
- Nail polish solvent
- Nail repair cement
- Nail repair tissue
- Nail strengthener
- Nail polish base coat
- Nail polish top coat
- Selection of coloured nail polishes
- Quick drying spray
- Client record cards

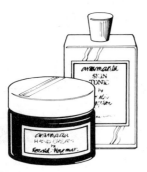

THE MANICURE

While a manicure is being performed the client should sit comfortably with her arms supported by a small table or manicure trolley. The manicurist should sit directly opposite the client. If this is not possible, a small cushion placed on her lap will help to support the arm.

Check both of the client's hands for any sign of a contra-indication. If there is any sign of infection the manicure should not be performed.

Discuss with the client what length and shape she would like her nails to be. Ask the client to choose the type and colour of nail polish that she requires.

Nail Shapes

The shape of one's nails is a personal consideration. Some clients like to have very long, brightly coloured nails. Others (especially men) may wish to have short or unpolished nails.

The shape of the nails should suit the shape of the hand. Small, dainty hands look better if the nails are filed moderately short in a slight oval. A light colour would enhance their delicate nature.

An oval hand is the ideal shape. The long, oval nail may be painted in any colour. The nails may be enhanced if the lanula is left free of colour.

The medium to broad hand often has wide nails. The nails look better if they follow the shape of the fingertips and are not pointed. They look best when shaped to a moderately short length and painted with a dark polish. A narrow line at each side may be left free of colour to make the nail appear slimmer.

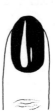

Small nail

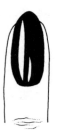

Oval nail

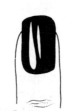

Medium nail

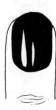

Square nail

The larger, square hand usually has wide, square nails. Do not file to a point but follow the shape of the fingertips. Leave a narrow, uncoloured strip down each side and paint with a dark nail polish.

It is very important that all equipment and instruments are cleaned and sterilised every time they are used.

The equipment and materials should all be kept together either on a special trolley or in a tray or basket. They can be moved easily to wherever they are required.

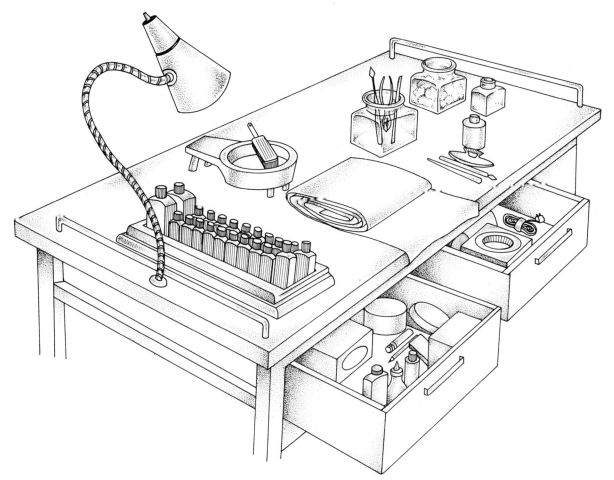

Each step of the manicure should follow a set pattern. The thumb should be worked on first, followed by the little finger, then the ring and middle fingers and finally the index finger.

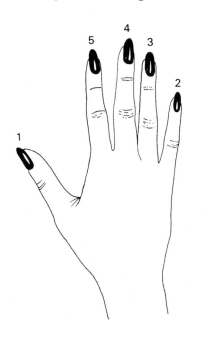

By following this pattern the manicurist will automatically know which finger to work on next. It also reduces the accidental touching of nails once polish has been applied to them. This same pattern should be followed throughout the manicure from the removal of the old polish, shaping, cuticle work, hand massage and applying of the new polish etc.

Method

1 Remove the client's rings, watch and any jewellery, and place them in a small bowl. Turn back the client's sleeves to above the elbow if possible.

2 Ask the client if she is right or left-handed. Thoroughly inspect the hands for signs of lack of care. If the client is right-handed, commence work on the left hand. By doing this, the right hand will have a chance to soak longer and so the tissues will soften. If the client is left-handed, work on the right hand first.

3 Apply an antiseptic solution to a cotton-wool pad and wipe it over the client's hands.

4 Apply nail polish remover to a pad of cotton-wool. Hold one end of it between the index

finger and middle finger and the other end between the ring and little fingers. This makes a firm pad under the ring and middle fingers. Support the underside of the client's fingers.

5 Place the pad on the nail to be worked on and gently rock it from side to side. This will dissolve the old nail polish. Slide the cotton-wool pad from the cuticle to the tip of the nail to remove the polish. Repeat the procedure for each finger of both hands using the set pattern. If a dark polish is being removed more than one cotton-wool pad may be required. Some people prefer to use a new pad for each finger.

6 Wrap cotton-wool around the end of an orange stick and apply some more nail polish remover. Gently wipe the cotton-wool along the cuticle and nail walls to remove any remaining polish.

7 For a right-handed person, shape the nails of the left hand following the set pattern. Use a long, flexible emery board. Always file in one direction, from the sides of the nail towards the tip. Do not use a sawing action as this will split the nail. Do not file too low at the sides as this can cause a hangnail. When the correct shape has been achieved, bevel the free edge of the nail by drawing the emery board over the free edge. This will avoid splitting and remove any roughness.

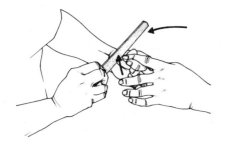

8 Apply cuticle cream with an orange stick to the base of each nail of the first hand. Massage it well into the cuticle with fingers and thumbs working together.

9 Soak the client's fingers in a bowl of warm soapy water.

10 While the left hand is soaking, shape the nails of the right hand. Apply cuticle cream to the right hand.

11 Remove the left hand from the water and dry it. Soak the right hand in the soapy water.

12 Wind a small wisp of cotton-wool around the end of an orange stick, then dip this into cuticle remover. Work gently in a circular movement around the edge of the cuticle and nail wall, easing it back. This will loosen the cuticle and dislodge any remaining tissue or dirt.

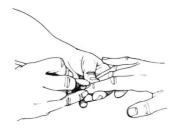

Some manicurists like to use a cuticle knife. It must be kept wet by being dipped into water before use on each nail. Any dead tissue adhering to the nail can be removed by gently moving the knife in a circular movement. To avoid scratching the nail or damaging the cuticle, the knife must be used flat, in a horizontal position to the nail, not pointing at an angle to it.

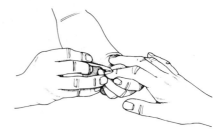

13 Dip a nail brush into water, then brush back towards the cuticle. This also helps to push the cuticle back as well as removing any cuticle remover that may be on the nail.

14 Dry the nails with a tissue, gently easing back the cuticle.

15 Use a dry, rubber hoofstick on the nails. Work gently in a circular movement all around and just under the nail wall and cuticle. This will stimulate the tissues under the nail as well as pushing back the cuticle.

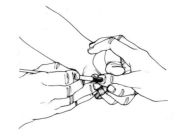

16 Remove any loose cuticle or hangnail with dry cuticle clippers. If there is any dry skin at the side of the nails, remove it with a pumice stick.

17 Check the edges of the nail and lightly file with an emery board if necessary.

18 Apply a little hand cream or lotion to the hand and wrap it in a towel.

Repeat the same procedure on the other hand.

Hand Massage

Repeat each massage movement four times. The hand and arm should be supported at all times. Spread hand cream or lotion over the hand and arm.

Method

1 Perform an effleurage over the hand and arm.

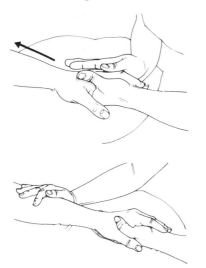

2 Work hand cream all around the elbow using a friction movement.

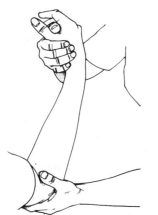

3 Perform a sliding friction with the thumbs, working up the centre of the arm (between the radius and the ulna) from the wrist to the elbow.
4 Perform petrissage around the wrist in 4 places.

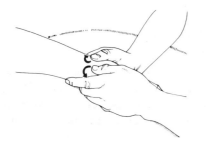

5 Hold the client's wrist with one hand. Lock your hand with the client's hand. Stretch the client's wrist by pulling the hand straight forward. Keep the tension and flex the hand back, then relax it. Keep the locked position and rotate the wrist both ways.

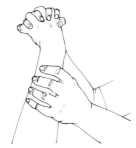

6 Slide the thumbs in a friction movement between the metacarpals on the back of the hand. Work from the phalanges to the wrist. Work across the back of the hand.

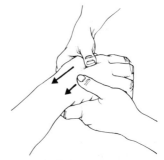

7 Rotate each finger both ways. Stretch the joints by pulling forward, holding the finger below the first joint.

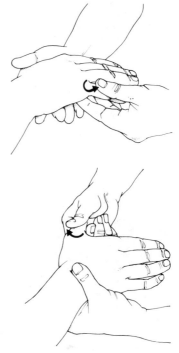

8 Turn the hand so that the palm is uppermost. Perform friction with the thumbs over the palms of the hand.

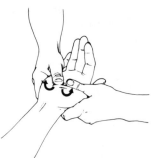

9 Slide your hands over the client's hands. Start with your fingertips over the client's fingertips. Slide up the hand, palm over palm. Slide down the thumb, grasping it gently.

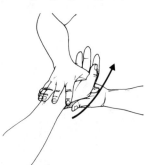

10 Hold the client's thumb in one hand and the little finger with the other. Shake the hand quickly and rhythmically, rolling it between your own hands.

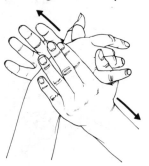

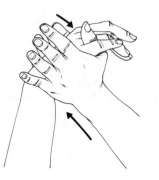

11 Perform an effleurage over the back of the hand and arm. Smooth off any excess cream.
12 Repeat on the other hand.
13 Wipe over the nails of both hands with a cotton-wool pad soaked in nail polish remover to remove any oil. Rinse off in water and dry the hands thoroughly.
14 The nails are now ready for buffing. If no polish is being applied a buffing paste or powder is used. The chamois buffer is brushed across the nail in one direction only. No buffing paste or powder is used if polish is to be applied.

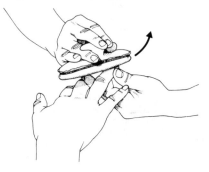

Nail Repairs

Method

1 Wipe over the nail with nail polish remover. Tear off a small piece of the special tissue supplied with the nail repair kit. It should be slightly larger than the area of torn nail.
2 Apply liquid cement to the tissue.
3 Use an orange stick to place the tissue, cement side down, onto the torn nail so that part of it overlaps the free edge. Use the orange stick to make sure that the tissue is not wrinkled and to tuck the tissue underneath the free edge. Make sure that the tissue is firmly stuck to the nail.
4 Smooth off any unevenness using solvent on an orange stick or even with your thumb.
5 When the repair is thoroughly dry, apply a base coat, nail polish and top coat as required.

Nail Painting

Work on the nails in the same set pattern used for the manicure.

The bottles of base coat and polish must be held between the thumb and index finger. The client's fingers can then be supported with the remaining fingers. If a nail strengthener is used, apply it before the base coat.

Method

1 Apply a base coat to the nails of both hands. It should be applied in three or four light strokes, brushing from the cuticle to the nail tip. It may also be applied with one stroke across the nail, followed by three strokes up to the nail tip. Care must be taken not to use too much base coat or polish otherwise the cuticle will be 'flooded'. The purpose of a base coat is to even out any ridges and to give a smooth surface for the coloured polish. It also protects the nail from the staining caused by some dark polishes.

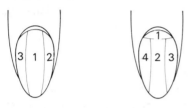

2 If any base coat or nail polish gets onto the cuticle or has flooded it, dip a plain orange stick into nail polish remover and stroke it across the unwanted polish.
3 Allow the base coat to dry. Touch the very tip of the first thumb to test if it is dry. Do not apply the next coat until the previous one is completely dry or it will flake off.
4 Apply the first coat of nail polish in the same manner as the base coat. Allow it to dry thoroughly.
5 Apply a second coat and allow it to dry thoroughly.

The nail polish should be applied very thinly. It is better to apply three thin coats than two thick coats. The thicker the coats, the longer they take to dry. Polish is more likely to chip if it is applied too thickly.

If a cream-type polish is used, a top coat should always be applied. It is not deemed necessary to apply a top coat over frosted or pearlised nail polish, though some people prefer it. If necessary, apply a quick drying spray, directing the spray away from the client.

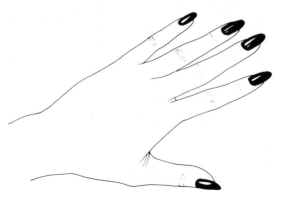

French Polish

In this method of painting the nails, a layer of white nail polish is applied around the nail tip. A pale pink polish is used for the main part of the nail.

Nail Design

Some clients like to have a design applied to their nails. Use one or several colours. Gold or jewellery stones may also be stuck onto the nails.

Hand and Nail Treatments

Simple Oil Treatment

A simple method is to soak all the fingernails in warm olive or almond oil for ten to fifteen minutes. Blot off any surplus oil and gently ease the cuticles back.

Heated Oil Treatment

This is very useful for fragile or damaged nails.

Method

1 Apply a liberal amount of oil to the nails. Bind them lightly in a cotton bandage. Apply further oil so that it soaks in.
2 Have a trolley ready with a towel covering a cushion on top. Rest the client's hand upon it. Apply infra-red heat to the fingers for 5–10 minutes. Protect the rest of the hands with a towel in case they get too warm.
3 At the end of the time, switch off the lamp and remove the bandages. Massage any remaining oil gently into the area around the nail. Blot off any surplus oil.
4 Gently ease back the cuticle with a wisp of cotton-wool on the thicker end of an orange stick. Do not remove the last traces of oil from the nails with nail polish remover. Do not apply nail polish.

Salt Treatment

Make a loose paste of household salt in olive oil. Massage this paste over the skin of the hands and elbows, if necessary, for 5 minutes. Use gentle friction movements. This will improve the circulation and remove any dry loose skin cells. Blot off the oil and wipe over the area with a skin freshener, or better still, the inside of a lemon.

Bran Treatment

Make a loose paste of bran, olive oil and a little lemon juice. Rose water may be used instead of lemon juice if the skin is very dry.

Massage the paste over the hands and wrists. Leave to soak in for 10 minutes. Wash off with warm water and dry thoroughly.

Paraffin Wax Treatment

This treatment is especially beneficial for clients who suffer from rheumatic conditions. It is also very useful for people who perform hard manual work, such as gardeners, whose hands have become cracked and ingrained.

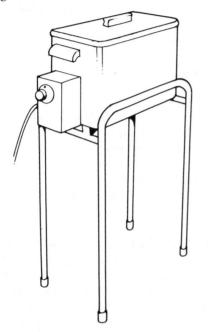

Paraffin wax heater

Method

1 Soak the hands in warm water. If the hands are very ingrained, make up a solution of Epsom salts.
2 Dry the hands thoroughly.
3 Apply several layers of wax to the hands and wrists. The wax should be as hot as the client can comfortably stand. It can be applied either by dipping the hand several times into a special bath or with a brush.
4 Wrap the hand in a polythene bag. Then wrap it in a towel to keep it warm.
5 Repeat on the other hand.
6 Leave the hands wrapped for approximately 15 minutes or until the wax is opaque and the heat has been expended.
7 Remove the wax.
8 Apply a light oil and give a hand massage. If required, give a manicure in the usual manner.

ARTIFICIAL NAILS

There are several different types of artificial nails:
   simple stick-on false nails
   silk wrap
   nail extensions (sculptured nails).

Artificial nails should not be applied to any fragile or pitted nails or when the surrounding skin is inflamed or damaged.

Simple Stick-on False Nails

This type of nail has been available for many years. They are often bought by the client for self-application. This type of nail is not permanent, lasting for only one or two days. It is inadvisable to keep them on for longer than forty-eight hours.

Select nails nearest in size to the client's own nails for shape and size. If too long or too wide, they may be paired down slightly so as to correspond to the client's own nails. Manicure the client's hands, but do not apply any base coat etc.

Method

1 Make sure that the client's nails are free from any grease by wiping with a nail polish remover that does not contain any oil.
2 Slightly roughen the underside of the false nail with an emery board to ensure maximum adhesion. The false nails may be softened by placing them in warm water for a few minutes. They must be thoroughly dried before application.
3 Apply a small amount of adhesive to the edges of the client's nail and to the underside of the false nail. Allow it to dry for a couple of minutes.
4 Slide the false nail flat along the client's nail until it just touches the cuticle. Shape it around the nail. Hold it in place for one minute, making sure that the edges adhere together.
5 Use an orange stick dipped into nail polish remover to remove any excess adhesive.
6 Repeat the procedure individually on each nail. Allow the adhesive to dry completely for about 10 minutes.

Apply nail polish in the usual manner.

The nails can be removed by softening the adhesive with an oil-based, acetone-free, nail polish remover. Many nails can be dissolved by acetone, so do not use any nail polish remover containing this. The false nails may be gently lifted from the nail with an orange stick. If the old adhesive is thoroughly cleaned from the false nail, it may be re-used by the client.

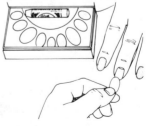

Silk Wrap

This technique is very similar to the way nails are mended with tissue. Pieces of very fine silk are cut to the same size as the nail.

Nail glue is applied to the nail. The silk is eased onto the nail. This is then covered with two or three layers of the special glue. Each layer should be allowed to dry before applying the next layer. The nail is then buffed smooth until it is transparent.

Nail polish may then be applied.

Nail Extensions (Sculptured Nails)

There are several techniques for applying nail extensions. An acrylic substance may be used. Other techniques use a gel or even fibreglass. Some require 'curing' with ultraviolet light, others do not. Some only require a nail tip while others need a full plate for the extension. The different manufacturers advocate their own specific methods.

Acrylic Nails

1 Gently buff the natural nail with a special emery board to roughen it. This will provide a good key for the acrylic mixture.
2 Thoroughly cleanse and disinfect the nail.
3 Apply a shaped nail tip over the tip of the natural nail to form a bed for the acrylic paste. Buff the natural nail to give better holding for the paste.
4 Mix the acrylic powder with the liquid to form a smooth paste.
5 Apply the paste evenly over the natural nail and nail tip with a good quality brush. Sable is often used.
6 Carefully build up the thickness of the acrylic nail, shaping it as you do so. Take care not to get it onto the cuticle.
7 When the acrylic is dry, file the new nail into shape.
8 Buff the nail so that there are no rough areas.
9 Apply nail polish.

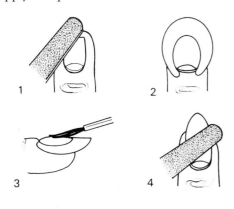

Gel Nails

The natural nail must be thoroughly disinfected and buffed to roughen it.

Apply the gel over a nail tip. Some types need to be 'cured' under an ultraviolet light. Other gels are 'cured' by the use of a spray. You can then shape, buff and paint the nails.

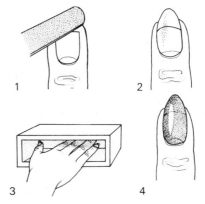

Fibreglass Nails

This newer technique is a very simple method of applying a fine layer of resin. It may be applied directly to the nail or over a nail tip if preferred. The natural nail does not need to be roughened and the natural oils are not removed so that the nails do not dry out. These nails are easily removed by soaking in a mixture of acetone and cuticle oil for about twenty minutes.

Common Problems Found with False Nails

Broken Nails

Either the nails were too long for the client to cope with or the acrylic or gel was too thin.

Nails Coming Off

Either the natural nail was too smooth because it was not buffed sufficiently or the nail has caught on something.

Nail Lifting at the Edges

Either the natural nail was not buffed sufficiently at the edges or was not free of oil before the nail was applied. Occasionally clients 'pick' at a new nail which can cause it to lift or break off.

Nails Become Yellowish

This is often because the client has not used a base coat under a dark polish. Smoking can also cause nails to turn yellow.

Cuticles Become Inflamed

This is either due to poor manicure technique or the client may be allergic to the ultraviolet.

General Infection

The nail was not sufficiently disinfected.

PEDICARE

A good pedicare will help to nourish the tissues and improve the circulation. The massage will stimulate the foot and leg muscles and discourage chilblains.

A pedicare is performed in a very similar manner to a manicure. The materials required are the same as for a manicure (pages 129–30) with the addition of a footbath, antiseptic and hard skin remover.

Method

1 Soak both feet in a bath to which antiseptic has been added.
2 Remove any hard skin with a hard skin remover.
3 Remove the feet from the footbath and dry thoroughly.
4 Remove the old nail polish from both feet and wrap one foot in a towel.
5 Shape the nails with the strong side of an emery board. File across the nail towards the tip from each side. Do not file backwards and forwards or the nail will split. The nails should not be curved, nor should they be taken too low at the sides or they will become ingrowing. If necessary use scissors or nail clippers first.

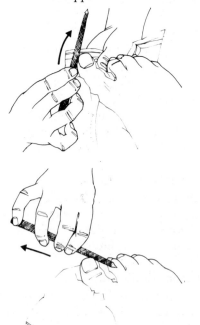

6 Apply cuticle cream. Massage it well into the skin all around the nail.
7 Wrap the first foot in a towel.
8 Shape the nails of the other foot and apply cuticle cream.
9 Work now on the first foot. Wrap a wisp of cotton-wool around an orange stick. Apply cuticle remover to the cotton-wool. Work around the cuticle in a circular manner, gently loosening them and pushing them back.

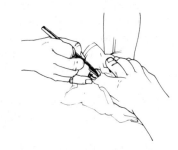

10 Gently loosen all the dead tissue around the cuticle with a cuticle knife. Make sure that it is kept wet by frequently dipping it in water.

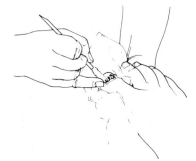

11 Dip a nail brush into water. Brush it over the nails to push the cuticle back.
12 Dry the nails and press them back with a tissue.
13 Use a dry hoof stick to push the cuticle back.

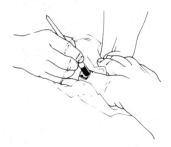

14 Remove any loose cuticle with clippers.

15 Wrap the foot in a towel and repeat the procedure on the other foot.
16 Massage both feet and legs.
17 Wipe over all the toenails with nail polish remover to remove any oil.
18 Place tissues or disposable pads between the toes to keep them separated.
19 Apply a base coat.
20 Apply two or more coats of nail polish. Allow them to dry thoroughly before applying the next coat.
21 If a cream nail polish is used, apply a top coat.
22 Remove the toe dividers when the nail polish is dry. A quick drying spray may be used to hasten the process.

Massage for Pedicare

Method

1 Apply a foot cream to the foot and leg as far as the knee.
2 Perform an effleurage up to the knee.

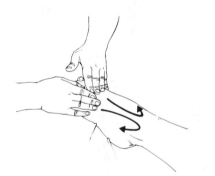

3 Perform petrissage around the ankle in four positions.

4 Support the leg above the ankle and rotate the foot each way.

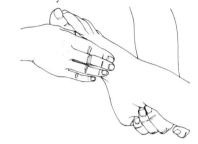

5 Perform a friction movement with the thumbs between the metatarsals, working upwards from the toes to the ankle.
6 Fan the toes and extend them upwards.
7 Perform frictions with the thumbs on the soles of the feet. Care must be taken that this does not cause irritation to the client.
8 Perform frictions around the heel.
9 Ask the client to keep the foot firm and work your hands briskly in a friction movement up the back of the leg.

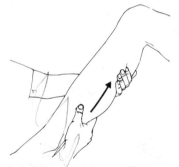

10 Finish the massage with an effleurage.
11 Remove any surplus cream and wrap the foot in a towel.
12 Repeat the same procedure on the other foot.

Many people like to apply a light dusting of talcum powder to the feet to complete the treatment.

Chapter 15

Hair Removal

Most women living in a 'Western' culture wish to have hair removed from their bodies at some period in their lives. For causes of hair growth see Chapter 9.

There are two main methods of removing hair: *epilation/electrolysis* and *waxing*.

EPILATION/ELECTROLYSIS

The removal of hair by the use of an electrical treatment is the only permanent method. There are three forms of this treatment:

1 galvanic
2 diathermy
3 blend.

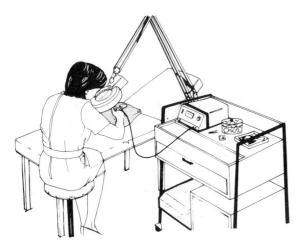

Work position

Galvanic Method

This is the oldest method of hair removal. It is referred to as *electrolysis*. However this term has now become the generic name for all forms of electrical hair removal of a permanent nature.

Galvanic electrolysis uses a direct electrical current. In order to complete the electrical circuit, the client holds a bar covered with an absorbent material that has been soaked in saline. The bar is connected to the positive terminal of the galvanic equipment. The needle holder is connected to the negative terminal.

The needle is inserted along the underside of the hair into the follicle. The needle is held in the follicle for $\frac{1}{2}$–2 minutes while the current is passing through it. The galvanic meter should never be higher than 2 milliamps.

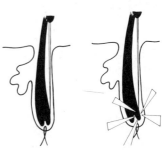

Correct   Electric current discharged here will destroy the hair

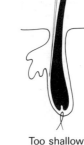 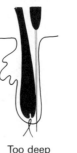 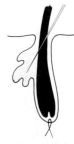

Too deep   Too shallow   Needle inserted into sebaceous gland

Needle insertion

The action of the direct current on the saline causes it to change the elements into entirely new substances. These are hydrogen gas, chlorine gas and sodium hydroxide (lye). This will act on the tissue adjacent to the needle where there is a natural moisture area, effectively 'killing' the hair growth. Although this is a slow method, many people still believe this is the most effective way to remove hairs.

Diathermy Method

This method uses a high frequency of 27.12 megahertz (MHz). Again, the needle is inserted into the hair follicle on the underside of the hair. The current is released either by a switch or button on the needle holder or by a foot pedal. The current creates an area of heat around the needle which effectively burns the root of the hair so that it will not re-grow.

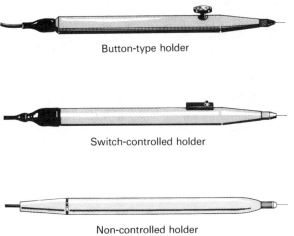

Button-type holder

Switch-controlled holder

Non-controlled holder
(for use with foot switch)

The time that the current is on is usually only one or two seconds, although there are variable factors.

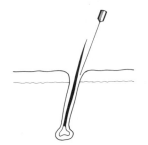

Correct needle insertion

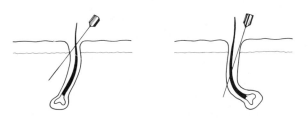

Incorrect needle insertions

The diathermy method is undoubtedly the fastest method of permanent hair removal. In some instances it may cause discomfort.

Blend

The blend machine uses a combination of the galvanic and the high-frequency currents. A greatly reduced intensity of current is used for approximately 5 seconds. The lye is still produced in the tissues around the needle. The area heated by the high-frequency current helps to disperse the lye in a wider area than when just the galvanic current is used.

Tweezer Method

This method uses tweezers to conduct a high-frequency current to the shaft of the hair. In theory the current is supposed to travel down the hair to the bulb and coagulate it. It is certainly a painless method but takes up to two minutes for each hair to have any effect.

Sterilisation

All instruments must be thoroughly cleaned before they are sterilised.

Needles

These may be purchased in pre-sterile packs. Re-usable needles must be sterilised in a bead steriliser for 20 minutes once the steriliser has reached its operating heat.

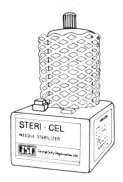

Bead steriliser

Forceps and Chucks

These may be sterilised by placing them in a liquid steriliser for 30 minutes. They must then be rinsed in running water to remove all the sterilising fluid. Care must be taken to see that this does not get onto the skin. The forceps are then clean but not sterile. Alternatively, they may be placed in an autoclave for 30 minutes.

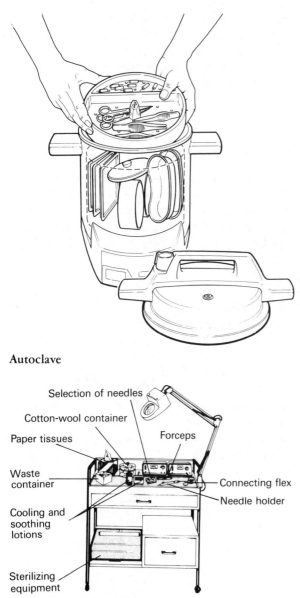

Autoclave

Selection of needles

Cotton-wool container

Paper tissues

Forceps

Waste container

Connecting flex

Needle holder

Cooling and soothing lotions

Sterilizing equipment

A typical trolley layout

It is generally considered that cotton-wool, tissues etc. need not be sterile but must be freshly taken from their container.

DEPILATORY WAXING

There are two types of wax that the professional may use: *warm wax* or *hot wax*. A cold or cool wax is available but is only used by the inexperienced person or by members of the public.

Wax may be used to remove hair from the legs, the bikini area, under the arms, the abdomen, the back and the face.

Antiperspirants, deodorants or perfumed talcum powder should not be used over the area for twelve hours following waxing.

Warm Wax

This is a very effective method for removing unwanted hair. The wax is heated in a special container until it is the consistency of runny honey. It should be warm when applied to the skin, not hot. Different manufacturers advocate the most effective temperatures for their own products. Warm wax is totally hygienic because it is not re-usable. It is much less painful to use than hot wax and is far easier to clean from the skin after use. Warm wax does not smell nearly as unpleasant as hot wax.

Contra-indications

　　Skin that is broken through, cuts or abrasions
　　Bruises
　　Skin infections, boils, rashes etc.
　　Varicose veins
　　Very thin or delicate skin
　　Ultra-sensitivity
　　Moles, warts
　　Before or after electrolysis or ultraviolet treatment
　　to that area

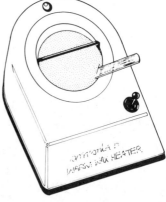

Warm wax heater

Hair should be at least ½ centimetre long before it can be removed effectively with warm wax. Growth will take 2–6 weeks depending on how fast the hairs grow.

The couch should be protected with heavy polythene sheeting. A sheet of couch roll should be placed on top for the client to sit on. Some people also like to protect the floor with polythene.

Method

The wax should be heated prior to the client's arrival. Some waxes take longer to heat than others, as do heaters.

You will need fabric cut into suitable lengths and widths. This is very much a personal choice. Strips can be long or short, narrow or wide according to preference. Pre-cut strips may also be purchased.

Protect the client's clothing with paper napkins.

Method

1 Wipe the skin with a strong antiseptic lotion to remove any oils, dead skin cells or local bacteria. Allow this to dry.
2 Apply unperfumed, plain talc to the area. This will absorb any moisture and keep the skin dry so that the wax will coat the hairs, not the skin.
3 Dip a wooden disposable spatula into the wax. Wipe the underside of it free of wax so that it will not drip.
4 Apply a very thin film of wax in the direction of the hair growth. Remember that not all hair grows in the same direction. The wax strip should be 40–50 mm (1½–2 inches) wide with straight, even edges.
5 Press a strip of fabric onto the wax and rub firmly so that all the wax adheres to the fabric.
6 Lift the lower end of the fabric. Hold the skin taut. With a quick movement, pull the fabric in an upward movement as near the skin as possible. Do not pull outwards from the skin as this will stretch it. Pull against the direction of the hair growth.

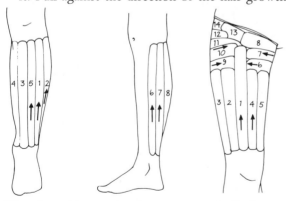

Direction of long strips for warm wax depilation

7 As soon as the strip is removed, rub the area with the flat of the hand. This will help considerably to stop the stinging sensation.
8 If some of the hairs remain, they may be waxed a second time. If there are only one or two hairs, they may be removed with tweezers. Apply the next wax strip and continue.

The strips of fabric may be used a number of times until they are coated with wax.

The area just outside the central line of the front of the lower leg is usually less sensitive than the inner aspect. Remove as much hair from the front and sides of the leg as possible before turning the client over. The client will often be more sensitive when she cannot see what is happening.

When waxing is completed, any wax remaining on the skin may be removed with massage oil. Very occasionally this may cause a slight irritation. Remove the oil with a tissue and clean the area with an antiseptic spirit solution.

Apply a soothing antiseptic lotion if the skin is at all reddened or dry.

For bikini line, underarm and facial waxing the wax must be put on in much smaller strips. The skin must be kept taut. If convenient, the client may be asked to help hold the skin. If waxing is performed on the face it must be used very carefully.

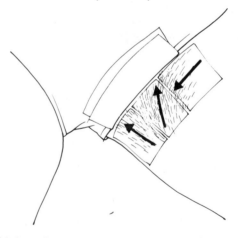

Bikini waxing

If the hair does not come out in these areas, only apply wax once more as the skin can become very tender.

Occasionally spots of blood may appear. The area must be very carefully cleansed with an antiseptic lotion. The strips and cleansing material must be very carefully disposed of. The therapist must also thoroughly clean her own hands with an antiseptic lotion. If the therapist has any cuts or abrasions on her hands, these must be covered with a plaster before commencing waxing.

For hygienic reasons, heat only enough warm wax for that client's treatment. Any wax remaining after use should be thrown away. Disposable spatulae should be used at all times. The wax container must then be thoroughly cleaned. Alternatively, a new disposable spatula may be used *every time* that wax is taken from the heater and applied to the skin.

Hot Wax

This is a rather old-fashioned type of waxing. It is banned completely in North America for hygienic reasons. The best depilatory wax is made from beeswax and oils. The wax should always be heated in a thermostatically controlled heater. On no account should it be heated over a direct flame.

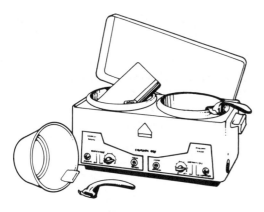

Dual pan (hot wax) heater

Any wax will deteriorate if overheated. There is always the danger of it catching fire if the heat is not fully controlled.

Because of modern hygiene regulations, wax should *never* be re-used. It is quite impossible to sterilise hot wax. Straining the wax does not eliminate bacteria and dead skin cells. It would need to be fast-boiled at 95 °C (203 °F) for 30 minutes to kill any bacteria in it, and this would damage the wax. Normal hot wax heaters will not heat to this temperature. Disposable spatulae must always be used.

Contra-indications
These are the same as for warm wax (page 142).

Method
Protect the couch with polythene sheeting. Place a sheet of couch roll on top for the client to sit on. Protect the client's clothing where necessary.

The wax should already be heated. Test the temperature of the wax on your own wrist before using it on the client.

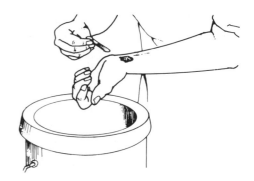

Testing temperature

1 Cleanse the area with a spirit solution to remove dead skin cells and natural oils. Allow it to dry.
2 If working on the leg, apply the wax in several strips about 5 cm (2 inches) wide and of a convenient length. Some people like a short strip of 10 cm (4 inches) while others prefer strips of 20 cm (8 inches).
3 Apply the wax with a disposable spatula, first *against* the hair growth and then the other way, *with* the hair growth. The wax needs to be approximately 3 mm ($\frac{1}{8}$ inch) thick with a slightly thicker end. The edges should be straight and even.
4 Several strips may be applied at the same time, leaving a space between them for the next set of strips.

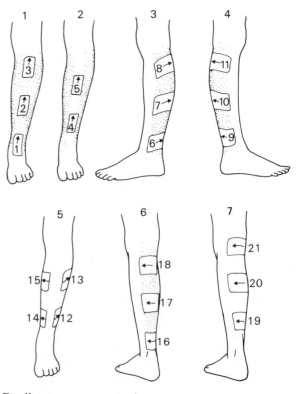

Depilatory sequence on legs

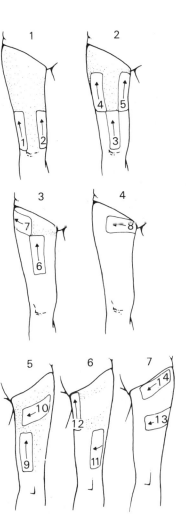

Depilatory sequence on thighs

5 When the wax has hardened it becomes opaque. Flick up the lower edge of the strip to facilitate its easy removal. Remove the strip quickly against the hair growth.

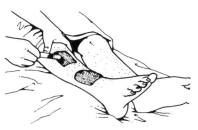

Apply strips

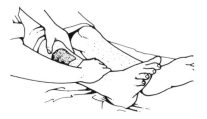

Press down wax

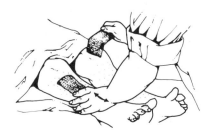

Take off strips, rub area

6 Quickly rub the area to reduce the stinging effect.
7 Repeat with the other strips, taking them off in the same order as they were put on.
8 Apply further strips of wax until all the hairs have been removed.

Hair does not always grow in the same direction. Care must be taken to see that wax is not applied across the direction of the hair growth.

Some hairs may be particularly stubborn. They may require a second waxing. If there are just one or two hairs they may be tweezed out.

When all the hairs have been removed from the front of the leg, assist the client to turn over. Repeat the process at the back of the leg.

At the end of the waxing all the wax must be removed with a spirit solution. A soothing antiseptic solution may then be applied.

OTHER METHODS OF HAIR REMOVAL

There are a number of alternative methods for removing air. They include:
    creams
    pumice
    razor
    plucking
    threading.

Creams

Depilatory creams dissolve hair at the level of the skin. The hair rapidly grows back as the root has not been treated. Some of the chemicals used may cause quite a severe skin reaction. This is not a professional method for removing hair. It is, however, favoured by members of the public.

Pumice

This may be a mitten made of a material rather like sandpaper, or an actual pumice stone. It is rubbed over the hairs in a circular fashion. It rubs the hair at the surface of the skin. The hair quickly regrows. Some of the skin surface may be damaged due to the harsh treatment. Again, it is only used by members of the public.

Threading

A thread of twisted cotton is rolled over the area where hair is to be removed. The hairs catch in the cotton and are pulled out, rather painfully. This skill is frequently practised by those of Indian or Mediterranean origin.

Razor

A razor is a quick and easy method of removing hair. The hairs are only removed at the level of the skin surface. They rapidly regrow and feel rather 'stubbly'. Frequently used by members of the public.

Plucking

This is only suitable for small areas such as the eyebrows. The forceps (tweezers) can be automatic or plain, either straight, round, slanted or pointed, long or short. Whichever design is chosen, they should be of a good quality and meet well at the tips.

Eyebrow Shaping

Method

1 Remove make-up on and under the eyebrows.
2 Wipe the forceps with a spirit or strong antiseptic. The forceps *must* be sterilised every time that they are used.

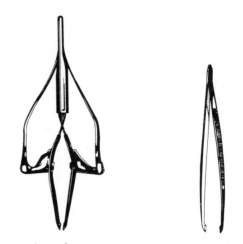

Automatic eyebrow tweezers   Tweezers

3 Wipe the eyebrow with cotton-wool and an antiseptic lotion. Wipe frequently during the procedure to remove stray hairs and to cool the area.
4 Gently stretch the skin between the second and third fingers.
5 Pluck in the direction of the hair growth. Do not snatch at the hair but gently ease it out.

Hair should be removed mainly from below the brow. Stray hairs between the brows and the temples may be removed as long as they do not form part of the main arch. Strong, long or discoloured hair in the brow may be removed as long as this does not alter the brow line.

Over-plucked or shaved eyebrows should be left and lightly trimmed regularly until a good shape is achieved. Remember to consult the client as to what sort of shape is required. For eyebrow shapes refer to Chapter 16.

Make-up

Make-up is a very ancient art. It is to be seen in the rock drawings of the primitive people of France, on early Chinese porcelain, Indian metalwork, Egyptian wall paintings and Italian mosaics. They all show that men as well as women made use of make-up. The kohl used by the Egyptians and the rouge used by Roman women are used in a similar way today.

Make-up is very much an art that can be learnt. In shops there is such an array of cosmetics that the untrained person can become quite confused. The therapist or beauty consultant should be familiar with what is new on the market so that clients can be best advised on what products to use.

Make-up should always look natural, though sometimes 'fashion' may say that harsher colours should be used to accentuate certain features. Make-up can be used to emphasise the good points or to hide weaker areas of a face. A light tone or highlighter will emphasise an area and a darker tone will shade it. If someone has a heavy jawline, a darker foundation or even a blusher blended over it will act as a camouflage. By emphasising the eyes one can draw the vision upwards and away from the jawline.

Many people believe that one can hide poor skin with heavy make-up. This is not so. A too-heavy make-up looks unnatural and shows up a blemished skin. The use of a concealer is much more effective.

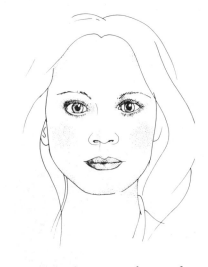

Last year's make-up fashion need not, of course, be the same as this year's. The therapist or beauty consultant must always take note of the client's wishes.

PREPARATION FOR MAKE-UP

Cleansing

Before the face is made-up, the skin must be thoroughly cleansed and the eyebrows tidied up. The shape of the face must be studied and any irregularities noted. The hairstyle should be taken into account as this can alter the visual shape of the face. If the make-up is for a special occasion it is necessary to ascertain the colour of the outfit. If the client is to be under artificial lighting this can alter the appearance of the make-up.

Ideally the client should be sitting in a comfortable chair in front of a mirror with a good white light which does not cast shadows. The hair should be held off the face with large hairslides.

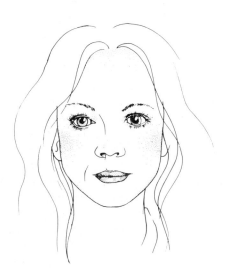

Moisturising

After cleansing and toning, a moisturiser must be applied to the whole face and throat. This will act as a barrier between the skin and atmosphere so that the skin will not become too dry. Some moisturisers will form a matte film and so prevent natural oils from seeping into the make-up.

Hygiene

When performing a make-up, always wash your hands before working on a client. Sterilise all the brushes, pencils etc. All the make-up products should be removed from their containers with a sterile spatula and placed onto a sterilised pallet. Any products left over must be discarded so as not to risk transferring infection or bacteria from one client to another.

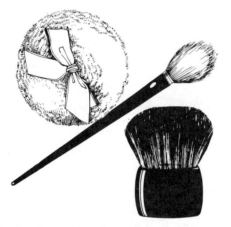

Powder brushes and puff

Cover Creams and Concealers

If there are any blemishes, broken capillaries, freckles, scars or dark tissue under the eyes, apply a cover cream or concealer and blend this over the area before applying the foundation. The foundation must be carefully applied so as not to dislodge the concealer.

APPLICATION OF MAKE-UP

Foundation

The foundation is applied next. It can be either a thin or thick liquid, a cream or a solid. In its simplest form it is a tinted powder made in a wide range of colours, held in a suspension of oil in water, or cream. Foundation is used to give an even tone to the skin, to cover freckles and broken veins.

For **dry, sensitive or mature skin** choose a foundation that is oil or cream-based.
For **oily or 'problem' skin** choose a water-based liquid foundation.
For **normal or combination skin**, a liquid or a solid foundation may be used.

Liquid foundation gives a better finish for day make-up unless the skin is badly blemished. It gives a lighter, more natural look. People who have allergic or hypersensitive skin should use products specially prepared for such conditions, containing as few known irritants as possible.

The therapist or beauty consultant should use a pallet to contain or mix the foundation before applying it to the client's skin. The colour to be applied should be near to that of the forehead of the client or just slightly lighter.

The foundation should only be applied to a small area of the face at a time because some foundations tend to dry rapidly. 'Dot' the foundation over the area and blend with a slightly damp, sterile natural sponge or dry latex sponge, using light, even strokes.

Powder

Powder is applied next. It is used to 'set' the foundation so that the make-up will stay fresh looking.

Powder can be tinted – which may alter the colour of the make-up, or translucent – which gives a matte finish without altering the colour of the foundation.

Powder may be loose or compressed. Professional make-up artists still use loose powder because it is more economical and colours can be mixed. It is easier to apply and produces a smoother finish.

Take sufficient powder for the face from the container and place on a tissue. Generously apply powder all over the face with a ball of cotton-wool, working from the neck upwards. Press the powder gently into the whole of the skin surface over the foundation. Where insufficient powder has been applied, the natural oils will quickly show through. Surplus powder should be removed using a large, soft, sterilised brush. Use a light movement in the direction of any hair growth, taking care not to brush the powder into any skin creases near the eyes or around the corners of the nose or mouth. If a more translucent effect is required, use a slightly dampened pad of cotton-wool to press onto the powder, taking care not to remove any of the make-up colour.

Blusher

A powder blusher is applied after face powder, a cream or liquid blusher is applied before powdering. The powder blusher is said to be the easiest to use. In some instances it may be advisable to apply a light covering of liquid blusher before powdering to show the facial outline and then powder blusher at the very end of the make-up.

The purpose of a blusher is to give the illusion of altering the contours of the face by accentuating or diminishing certain features. It adds warmth and colour.

Dark-coloured blushers can be used to create depth while light colours give prominence. Use them instead of highlighters and shaders which are often too hard for daytime make-up.

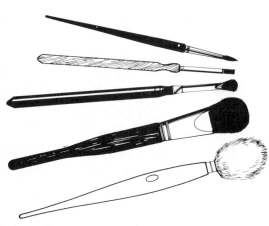

Make-up brushes

Face Shaping

On a young face with a good natural shape, apply blusher following the shape of the cheeks. On a more mature person with a good natural shape, apply blusher along the zygomatic arch so as to give greater prominence to the eyes.

There are some simple guidelines for applying the main colour blusher: apply blusher above an imaginary line from the corner of the mouth to the centre of the ear. No further in than the pupil of the eye. No lower than the nose and no higher than the eyebrow, at the side of the face.

The following points may be useful in correcting irregular features.

Square-shaped Face

Shade the corners of the face with darker blusher. Place a triangle of the main blusher on the cheeks to a level with the eyebrows. Lighten the centre of the forehead and chin. Arch the eyebrow shape.

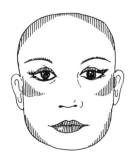

Round-shaped Face

Shade the sides of the face with darker blusher. Place a triangle of main colour blusher on the cheeks to the level of the eyes. Lighten the chin. Arch the eyebrows and shorten their length.

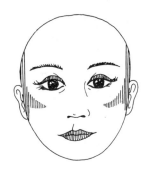

Rectangular-shaped Face

Shade around the hairline and the angles of the jaw with darker blusher. Place main colour blusher under outer corners of the eyes and out to the hairline. Lighten the tip of the chin. Shape fine, long eyebrows.

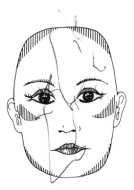

Triangular-shaped Face

Shade across the top of the forehead and the angles of the jaw with darker blusher. Place main blusher low on the cheeks and sweep upwards. Lighten the sides of the face and the chin. Shape long, fine eyebrows.

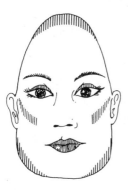

Diamond-shaped Face

Shade across the top of the forehead, the sides of the face and the chin with darker blusher. Place main blusher low on the cheeks and sweep upwards. Lighten the temples and angles of the jaw. Arch the eyebrows.

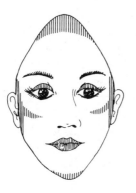

Heart-shaped Face

Shade along the sides of the hairline with darker blusher. Place main colour blusher across the cheeks. Lighten centre forehead and sides of cheeks. Gently arch the eyebrows.

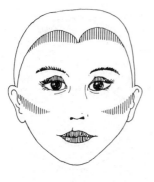

Chin

Where the jawline is squared or 'heavy', apply a darker shade of blusher to the corners of the face.

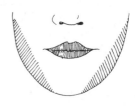

On a protruding chin, apply a darker blusher to the point of the chin. On a small or receding chin apply a lighter blusher or highlighter to the point of the chin.

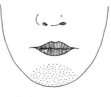

EYE MAKE-UP

Eyebrows

Ensure that the eyebrow shapes are correct for the shape of the face. Remove any straggling hairs before commencing the make-up (page 146).

If the eyebrows need lengthening or darkening this may be done with a brow pencil. Use short strokes in an upward movement towards the outer point. Then use a stiff eyebrow brush to soften the pencil strokes.

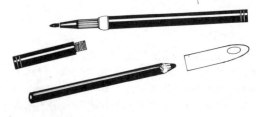

Eyebrow pencils

Eyeshadow

Eyeshadows may be in powder, gel, cream, or pencil form. They are available in a variety of colours and may be matte or pearlised, opaque or iridescent. Powder is the easiest form to use. It may be applied with a sterile brush or an applicator.

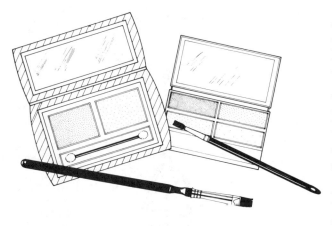

Take sufficient colour for both eyes from the container and place it on a pallet with a small spatula. On no account should a used brush or applicator touch the eyeshadows in their containers. Pencils should always be sterilised after use in an ultraviolet cabinet.

Remember that a light colour accentuates and draws out, while a dark colour gives depth. Eyeshadow emphasises the eyes and can change the whole look of the face.

The most usual method is to apply colour across the eyelids in bands. This can make the face look wider and eyes sometimes rather slit-like.

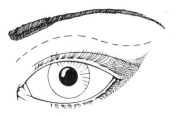

Eye make-up

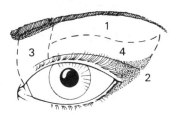

Alternative eye make-up

The following method of application is effective in making the eyes appear larger and giving a good proportion to the face.

Application of Eyeshadow

Begin by applying a light colour (highlighter) to the whole of the upper lid. Colours always need to be blended so that there are no hard lines.

To outline the eye, use a sterile eye pencil. Draw a line starting at the outer corner, for three-quarters of the way along the lower lid. Draw a thicker line, quarter of the way along the upper lid. Blend with an applicator.

Apply a third colour to the inner corner of the eyelid up to the eyebrow, blending inwards. It should be darker than the highlighting colour but lighter than the pencil applied at the outer corner.

The last colour should compliment the other colours used. Apply it to the centre of the eyelid, blending into the other three colours. The socket line will dictate how high you take it.

Great care must be taken to see that the delicate skin around the eyes is not stretched.

On completion, re-touch the colours if necessary. Check both eyes frequently for symmetry.

The following points may be useful for correcting irregular features of the eyes.

Prominent Eyes

Highlight under the brow and around the outer corner of the eyes. Use a deeper shadow across the lid.

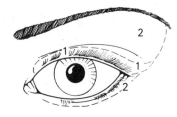

Small Eyes

Highlight under the brow using a light colour. Apply a pale shadow on the inner and outer part of the eyelid. Apply a darker shadow to the centre part of the eyelid.

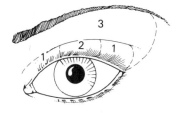

Overhanging or Drooping Eyelids

Highlight on the brow and on the inner corner of the eyelid. Apply a pale colour under the brow then a darker colour along the 'hanging' part of the lid. Finish with a deeper colour at the outer corner, winging it upwards and out.

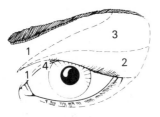

Close-set Eyes

Apply a pale colour to the brow and eyelid. Highlight under the centre of the brow. Apply a deeper colour over the lid and wing upwards.

'Bags' under the Eyes

Apply the foundation as normal then blend a lighter foundation over the 'bags'. For evenings, a white powder shadow may be used. Apply the eyeshadow in the normal way.

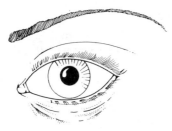

Eyeliner

This is one cosmetic which has a varying popularity depending on the dictates of fashion. It may be applied either just inside or outside the lash line. A new or sterilised applicator brush or pencil must be used.

False Eyelashes

False eyelashes are applied following eyeliner, if required.

Mascara

If necessary, an instrument for curling the lashes may be used before applying mascara.

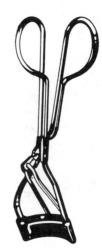

Automatic eyelash curler

The final stage of eye make-up is the application of mascara. It may be in block form, a cream or more commonly from a container with its own wand or brush. A new or sterile applicator should be used for each client.

Many mascaras are waterproof. They are available in a number of colours and shades – blues, greens, mauves, bronze, gold and the most popular, black. Some mascaras contain fibres to lengthen the natural lash. These should be used only by people who have no sensitivity or problems with their eyes.

Brush the lashes with a dry brush before applying the first coat to remove any powder. Use a dry brush to separate the lashes before applying further coats and on completion.

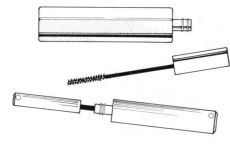

Mascara

Mascara should first be applied with a downward movement over the upper lashes. The underside of the lashes are then coated evenly. This is then repeated on the lower lashes. There must be no clogging. Finally all the lashes should be separated using a lash comb.

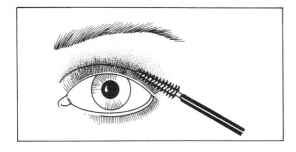

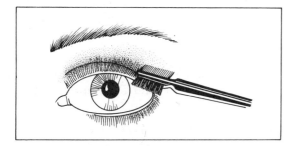

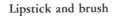

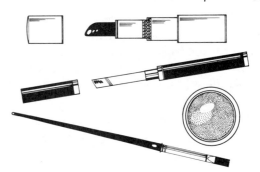

Lipstick and brush

To give greater staying power, lightly blot the lips and finely dust with loose powder before applying a second coat. Apply a lip gloss if required and check that the lips are symmetrical.

Natural-shape Lips
These are balanced both in width and depth.

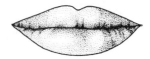

Full Lips
Draw a line with a lip pencil just inside the natural line. Fill in with lip colour.

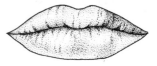

Thin Lips
Draw a line with a lip pencil just outside the natural line. Fill in with lip colour.

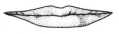

Uneven Lips or Lips Needing Correction
Draw the natural lip shape with a lip pencil. Fill in with lip colour, using a light shade for the smaller lip and a darker shade for the larger lip.

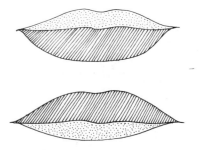

LIP MAKE-UP

Lipsticks may come as pencils, moulds, in stick or liquid form or as pressed powder. They may be of solid colour or opaque, cream, gloss or pearlised. They are made in a variety of colours from white to black, in varying shades of green, blue, mauve, yellow, pink or red.

The application of lipstick adds the final touch to the make-up. It completes the picture and balances it.

Lipstick should be placed on a pallet before being applied with a sterile brush. Outline the lips with a brush or lip pencil. The lips should be closed to give a firm surface to work on. Fill in the rest of the lip surface with a lip brush. Gently relax the lips and open the mouth to apply colour to the corners of the mouth. When applying lipstick, work from the outer corners of the lips inwards and then from the centre of the lips outwards.

Darker colours will make the lips appear smaller. Bright or light colours will enlarge their appearance. More than one colour may therefore be used to achieve the desired effect. Use a colour that tones with the blusher and compliments the foundation and the eye colours.

Lipstick with a blue tinge should not be used if the lips are at all blue themselves or if the client has a florid complexion.

At the end of the make-up, check that the whole face looks symmetrical and above all, natural. A soft look should be applied for daytime. A bolder make-up is used for evenings because artificial lighting may blanch make-up.

Remove the headband or slides and lightly dress the hair.

MAKING-UP DARK SKIN

The make-up for black or Asian skin will be slightly different from that used on light skin.

Applying Make-up

Care must be exercised when applying foundation, because the wrong shade (particularly one that is too pale) can make the skin look dull and grey. The great variety of skin colours and tones means that it is often easier to achieve a closer colour match by blending a foundation from two or more base colours. Any foundation should be near to the natural skin colour shade. Sometimes a dark skin may need only a covering of colourless gel rather than foundation.

When choosing blushers, use colours that emphasise and tone with the natural colour. The blusher should be non-greasy, preferably either a cream or gel. Powder blushers can dull the skin and do not adhere as effectively. If using face powder, this should be very fine and of a concentrated colour. White or colourless powders can also leave the skin looking grey and dull. Some people prefer not to use any powder at all.

Matte and cream eyeshadows with a higher wax content are particularly suitable, as these are more resistant to a slightly higher body temperature (page 26). The therapist should take advantage of the fuller range of colours that can be used to great effect, especially the more vibrant colours. When selecting eyeliner use eye pencils (kohl can be very effective) rather than liquid eyeliners which may streak.

Lipstick or gloss may be used on the lips, depending on the total look the client wishes to achieve. If using lipstick the richer colours are often the most flattering.

EYEBROW SHAPING

Eyebrows help to define and frame the eyes. Well-shaped eyebrows help to give an appearance of good grooming. Plucking the eyebrows is still considered to be the only reliable and safe method of shaping them. The use of creams or wax can damage the delicate tissues around the eye. A razor leaves sharp stubble hair. Electrolysis is expensive and will permanently change the eyebrows, which the client may wish to alter again at a later date.

Eyebrow shaping is partly governed by the shape of the face and partly by the dictates of fashion. Ideally the distance between the two eyes should be the width of one of them. If this is not the case, an illusion can be created by removing hairs at the inner aspect of the eyebrows to make the eyes appear less close together.

A **mature person** will probably look best with eyebrows shaped into a natural arch, neither left too thick nor plucked too finely.

A person with a **square-shaped face** will possibly look best with the eyebrows shaped to an angle just to the outside of the central line of the eye.

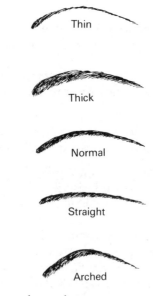

Different eyebrow shapes

The client with a **diamond or round-shaped face** should have the eyebrows arched in the centre.

The client with an **oblong-shaped face** should have the eyebrows plucked into almost a straight line.

Clients with a **triangular-shaped face** require a gentle arching in the centre of the eyebrow.

In selecting an eyebrow shape, the wishes of the client are of paramount importance.

Correct Length for Eyebrows

In order to determine the correct length for the eyebrows there are three main guidelines:
1 Place an orange stick beside the nose and the inner aspect of the eye. Any hairs on the inner side of the orange stick should be removed.
2 Place an orange stick in a line from the nose to the outer aspect of the eye. Remove any hair lying outside this line.
3 Place an orange stick in a line from the nose to the centre of the pupil of the eye. This is where the highest point of the arch should be.

Normally only hairs growing under the eyebrows are removed. However, a few stray hairs may also be removed from above to give a good line.

Contra-indications

Any eye disorders, e.g. stye, conjunctivitis
Any inflammation or swelling around the eye
Any cuts, abrasions or bruising

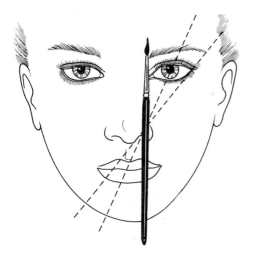

Method

Always use a good light when shaping the eyebrows. The forceps (tweezers) must meet well where they join (see page 146). They may be automatic or plain with either a straight, round, slanted or pointed head. The forceps must be sterilised beforehand.

1 Have the client sitting or lying in a comfortable position. Remove all make-up from on and just under the brow with cleansing milk and mild skin tonic. This is to remove any oils so that the forceps do not slip.
2 Define the shape and length that the eyebrows are to be.
3 Moisten pads of cotton-wool in warm water and apply to the eyebrows. This will help the tissues to relax so that the hairs will come out more easily. Repeat as necessary if the skin becomes sensitive.
4 Wipe the forceps with a spirit or antiseptic solution.
5 Gently hold the skin between the middle and index fingers, pressing slightly on the skin behind the hair. This can slightly 'deaden' the nervous sensation. Hold the hair firmly with the forceps and pluck it out in the direction of the growth.

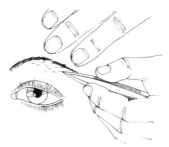

6 The hairs should be removed from the forceps by wiping them frequently on a pad of cotton-wool.
7 Some people prefer to work on each eyebrow alternately. Others prefer to complete one eyebrow before starting on the second eye. Check the shape frequently to make sure that they are symmetrical.
8 Wipe the eyebrows with an antiseptic solution and then brush them into shape.

Long hair may be trimmed with scissors if necessary. Discoloured hairs may be removed if they do not alter the brow line. Over-plucked, shaved or waxed eyebrows should be lightly trimmed at regular intervals until a good shape has been achieved.

Heavy brows should not be plucked to a fine line in just one session. Allow the client to get used to the gradual shaping. Remember to consult a client as to her wishes. You can always remove more hairs if required. You cannot compensate the client if you have removed too many.

EYELASH AND EYEBROW TINTING

Eyebrows help to emphasise facial expression. Eyelashes make a frame for the eyes. Permanent lash tinting will help to enhance the eyes and make the lashes look longer. It will also save the client from having to apply mascara daily. A tint will last as long as the lashes; about six weeks. Tints are available in black, brown, blue and grey.

Contra-indications

Any eye disorders, e.g. stye, conjunctivitis
Any inflammation or swelling around the eye
Any cuts, abrasions or bruising
A history of eye sensitivity or allergies

Patch Test

There are several makes of tint permitted under the EEC regulations. Before using any of them on a client a 'patch test' *must* be performed. A client may have a reaction to one brand but not to another. If you run out of the one that is normally used on a particular client, do not use another brand unless a patch test has been performed using that make.

A patch test should be performed 24–48 hours prior to tinting. It is easiest to test behind an ear where it will not show.

Cleanse an area behind one ear with surgical spirit. Apply a small amount of the tint (mixed according to manufacturer's instructions). Allow it to dry. Some people then cover the tint with collodian.

Check the area 24–48 hours later. If there is any sign of redness, irritation or inflammation, do not carry out a lash tint with this product. If the same reaction occurs with a tint produced by another manufacturer, advise the client against having lash tint at any future time. Any redness or irritation may be reduced by the use of calamine.

Requirements for Lash/Brow Tinting

Cleansing milk
Mild skin tonic
Assorted tint colours
10 volume hydrogen peroxide
Petroleum jelly
Eye shields
Cotton buds
Orange sticks
Spatulae
Tint brush (sterilised)
Cotton-wool pads (pre-shaped)
Tissues

Method for Tinting the Eyelashes

The client should be in a sitting or semi-recumbent position. Some clients prefer to be lying down. Discuss with the client which colour she wishes to have.

1 Cleanse around the eyes and eyebrows with cleansing milk. If required, the whole face can be cleansed. Make sure that the lashes are free of mascara. Use a mild skin tonic over the area to remove any oils.
2 Apply petroleum jelly, with an orange stick or applicator, in a line on both the upper and lower eyelids close to the lashes. Care must be taken not to touch the lashes, or the tint will not 'take'.
3 Place pre-shaped (half-moon) pads of damp cotton-wool under both eyes. Slide them in until they lie close to the lower lashes. Prepared paper eyeshields may be used instead.
4 Place the tint in a non-metallic dish. Mix into this the appropriate number of drops of 10 volume hydrogen peroxide. Be very carefully guided by the manufacturer's instructions.

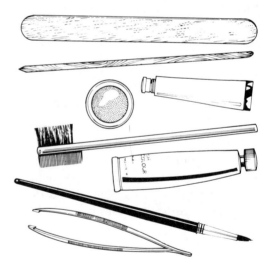

Lash tinting accessories

5 Apply the tint, using a sterile brush or an orange stick tipped with cotton-wool.
6 Ask the client to keep her eyes open. Apply the tint to both sets of lower lashes, working outwards from the roots to the tips.
7 Ask the client to close her eyes. Apply tint to both the upper lashes.
8 Cover the eyes with pads of damp cotton-wool. This assists the tinting process. It also helps the client to relax so that she will not open her eyes.

9 Test the colour after 5–15 minutes, depending on the manufacturer's instructions. When the desired tone has been reached, remove both the lower shaped pad and the top pad together from one eye. This should be done in a firm, even, rolling movement from the outer corner to the inner corner of the eye. This will remove most of the surplus tint. Remove the second pair of pads.

10 Remove any remaining tint with a rolled-up damp cotton-wool pad or cotton buds while the eyes remain closed.

11 Ask the client to open her eyes and check that no tint or petroleum jelly remains.

12 Apply a compress or damp cotton-wool pads to the eyes for five minutes to relax them.

13 When the eyelashes are dry, separate them with an eyelash comb.

Method for Tinting the Eyebrows

1 Cleanse the eye areas with cleansing milk and mild skin tonic.

2 Surround the eyebrows with a fine line of petroleum jelly.

3 Mix the tint with 10 volume hydrogen peroxide in a non-metallic dish. Two colours mixed together give a more muted colour, and in most cases a better appearance, than just using a black tint on its own.

4 Apply the tint first to the underlying hairs, lifting them up, and then to the top hair shaping the brow line. The tint can be applied with a fine, sterilised brush or an orange stick covered in cotton-wool.

5 Check the colour density after 2–3 minutes. If a deeper colour is required, leave on for a further 2–3 minutes. *Blonde hair* takes colour rapidly and overtinting will give a harsh appearance. *Red hair* may need longer to 'take' a tint. *Dark hair* will only require a little tint to even up the shading. Ensure that the tint is left on both brows for the same length of time. After the eyebrows have reached a satisfactory colour, remove the surplus tint with damp cotton-wool pads and/or a cotton bud. Make sure that none remains on the skin.

6 Make sure that all the petroleum jelly is removed.

7 Brush the eyebrows into shape.

8 If there is no sign of sensitivity, the eyebrows may now be shaped.

FALSE EYELASHES

These can be very effective for an evening or special event. They add length to short, straight lashes and supplement fine lashes, making them look longer and thicker.

There are two main types of false eyelashes: *semi-permanent individual lashes* and *strip lashes*.

Contra-indications

Any eye disorder, e.g. stye, conjunctivitis
Any inflammation or swelling around the eye
Sensitivity or reaction to the adhesive

If someone has a history of sensitivity or allergies, it is recommended that a skin test is performed 24–48 hours before applying false lashes.

Semi-permanent Individual Lashes

Individual lashes give a more natural look than strip lashes.

The client should be sitting up with her head supported but tilted slightly forward. Make sure the areas around the eyes are free of make-up and mascara. Select false lashes suitable for the client.

Method

1 Place a little of the special lash adhesive onto a small dish.

2 Pick up a lash with sterile forceps.

3 Dip the end of the lash into the adhesive so that it is coated just at the end.

4 Apply the false lash to the inner corner of the upper lid.

5 Slide the false lash down beside a natural lash until it rests as near to the eyelid as possible without touching it. Allow the adhesive to dry slightly before proceeding to the next lash.

6 Work towards the outer corner of the upper lid before proceeding to the lower lashes (if required).

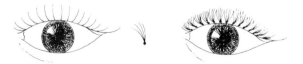

If watering occurs, ask the client to sit up and to gently blow her nose. This will drain fluid gently away from the eyes.

7 When the lashes have all been applied and are dry they may be curled using an eyelash curler (page 152). Eye make-up may then be applied.

Removal of Semi-permanent Individual Lashes

If left, the lashes will grow out with the natural lashes. However, sometimes they are required just for a special occasion and need to be removed afterwards.

1 The client should be sitting comfortably. Apply a special solvent to cotton-wool which has been wrapped around an orange stick.
2 Apply a little of the solvent to the base of the false lash.
3 When the adhesive has been softened the false lash may be gently slid up the lash until it can be lifted off. If the false lash does not slide easily, re-apply the solvent.
4 Gently remove all the lashes in this way. In some instances it may be easier to remove them in the reverse order to that of putting them on.

This type of false lash is not usually re-used by the client.

Strip Lashes

This type of false eyelash comes in matching pairs. They vary in shape, length and thickness. Some have a self-adhesive backing strip. Others require special adhesive.

Method

1 The client should be sitting comfortably. Measure the lashes to the width of the eye. Most lash strips need to be made shorter. Cut them at the end where the longest lashes are. These will be placed at the outer edge of the eye. Clip the lashes with scissors to give them a more natural appearance.

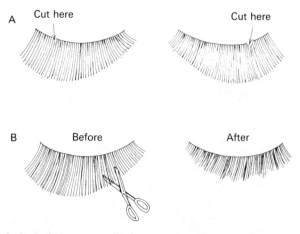

Strip lashes

2 Ask the client to close her eyes. Take hold of one strip with sterile forceps. Apply adhesive to the back of the strip.
3 Position the lash strip as close to the client's own lashes as possible without actually touching them.
4 Position the second strip and check that they are even. As the adhesive takes approximately three minutes to set, the strips may be carefully adjusted during this time if necessary.
5 When the adhesive has fully set, an eyelash curler may be used and eye make-up applied.

Removal of Lash Strips

1 To remove a lash strip, gently lift it up at the outer edge and peel it off the skin towards the inner corner of the eye.
2 Wipe the eyelid with damp cotton-wool.

These lash strips may be re-used by this client. They should be soaked in warm water and any adhesive gently removed. The clean lash strips should then be placed on a tissue and gently pressed dry. Roll this over a pencil so that the strips will retain their curled shape.

BLEACHING FACIAL HAIR

There are a number of proprietary brands of bleaching agents available. Always read their instructions before applying them. On no account should household bleach or plain hydrogen peroxide be used. It can burn and severely damage the skin.

The client should be reclining with her head back, or lying on a couch.

Method

1 Cleanse and tone the area. Make sure that it is thoroughly dry.
2 Mix the activating agents together in a non-metallic dish according to the manufacturer's instructions.
3 Use a small spatula to apply the mixture to the hair to be treated.
4 The mixture may be left in place for 5–15 minutes.
5 Check the colour after five minutes, then keep checking until the right degree of lightness has been obtained.

6 Remove the mixture by gently lifting with a thin spatula or by wiping with a tissue.
7 Rinse the area with warm water, using cotton-wool pads.
8 Dry the area and apply a light moisturiser.

Contra-indications
No irritation is commonly associated with this treatment but if it occurs, remove the mixture immediately. Do not apply to any area which has any blemishes or pustules, sensitive skin, or cuts or abrasions.

Chapter 17

Simple Cosmetic Formulae

Cosmetic chemistry is a very wide field. It takes many years to become an expert in order to understand how to use all the different ingredients. The therapist can only hope to touch on the subject, but should know a little about some of the materials used.

Included in this chapter are formulae published in *Harry's Cosmeticology*. However, difficulty may be experienced if you try to make up a professional formula as very few retail or wholesale outlets are able to supply the ingredients in small quantities. I have therefore also included a number of simple recipes using products easily obtained from a chemist and also some ordinary household products.

SOAP

The main constituents of soap are either fats or vegetable oils which are neutralised by an alkali. This may be potassium or sodium. Transparent soaps contain a glycerine or coconut oil. Many soaps contain a colouring agent and also perfume.

Some soap can prove too strong on facial skin, especially if this is at all sensitive. Unless thoroughly rinsed off, the alkali can cause dry patches to occur. Both the perfume compounds and the colour can cause an allergic reaction on some people. It is much better to freshen the face with warm water and to use a more effective method such as cleansing milk or cream.

DEODORANTS AND ANTIPERSPIRANTS

Bacteria occur naturally on the skin's surface. They grow more rapidly in a warm, moist atmosphere such as the axilla (underarm). When they start to break down the sweat and sebum in these areas this causes an unpleasant odour.

Deodorant

A deodorant, which may contain an antiseptic as well as a bactericide, will check the growth of bacteria. This will effectively remove the cause of the unpleasant odour.

Frequent washing with a mild soap will remove any stale sweat and decaying bacteria. Sodium bicarbonate has long been known to act chemically to destroy these bacteria. Some essential oils such as thyme also have a good effect as a bactericide.

Deodorant *(Harry's Cosmeticology)*	
	%
Hexamethylenetetramine	14.0–20.0
Zinc oxide	16.0–23.0
Starch	16.0–23.0
Petroleum jelly	38.0–43.0
Perfume	0.5–1.2

Antiperspirant

An antiperspirant, as the name implies, prevents the secretion of the sweat glands. Because of this, the bacteria do not grow so rapidly, therefore there is less decay to cause the unpleasant odour.

Antiperspirant *(Harry's Cosmeticology)*	
	%
Isopropyl myristate	32.0
Bentone 38	7.0
Ethyl alcohol	3.0
Zirconium hydroxychloride	47.0
Silicone	10.0
Perfume	1.0

TALC

Pure talc is used to absorb moisture on the body. It has a cooling effect as well as helping the skin to feel smooth. Talc should not be confused with talcum powder. Pure talc will normally make up only approximately 30 per cent of the ingredients of talcum powder. It should always be free of grit and alkali particles.

Talcum Powder *(Harry's Cosmeticology)*	
	%
Talc	75.0
Kaolin	10.0
Fumed silica	2.0
Magnesium carbonate	6.0
Zinc stearate	6.0
Perfume	1.0

DETERGENT CLEANSERS

These are made from modern synthetics such as petroleum derivatives and can be used in place of soap. In most cases they are very mild having a pH of 5.0–6.5, which is similar to that of the skin. They include soapless lather cleansers, which are particularly good for cleansing oily or blemished skin. They may have both an antiseptic and a germicidal agent added to them.

Germicidal Cleansing Gel *(Harry's Cosmeticology)*	
	%
Triclosan	3.0
Menthol	10.0
DEA-oleth-3 phosphate	2.5
Hydroxypropylcellulose	2.5
Amphoteric-1	5.0
Pure water	37.0
Ethanol (96%)	40.0

CLEANSERS

Cleansing Cream

There are over 100 formulae for cold creams including the one originally made by Galen for the women of ancient Greece. It is thought that cold creams got their name because first they had to be heated and then beaten until they were cold. It could also be because they feel cold on the skin when first applied. Traditionally they contained beeswax, oil of rose and olive oil or water. Modern cleansing creams contain mineral oil, beeswax, borax and water mixed to form an emollient. They are still normally perfumed with rose.

Cleansing cream should spread easily over the skin. Its melting point should be just lower than the skin's temperature so that it will melt quickly on touching the skin surface.

Cleansing cream will dislodge dead skin cells and dirt and dissolve make-up, making it easy to remove with a damp cotton-wool pad.

Cleansing Cream *(Harry's Cosmeticology)*	
	%
Beeswax	8.0
Mineral oil	49.0
Paraffin wax	7.0
Cetyl alcohol	1.0
PEG-15 Cocamine	1.0
Borax	0.4
Carbomer 934	0.2
Pure water	33.4
Perfume and preservatives may be added if desired.	

Cold Cream	
	%
Spermaceti	17.0
Beeswax	8.5
Almond oil	67.0
Glycerine	0.5
Single rose water	3.0
Rose or other essences may be added if desired.	

Cleansing Milk

These are usually an oil in water emulsion. They may contain ingredients such as cetyl alcohol, stearic acid or lanolin as well as mineral oil, spermaceti and water. They spread more easily and penetrate a little deeper than cleansing cream. They lift off dirt and dead skin cells but may take a little longer to remove make-up than a cleansing cream.

Cleansing Milk *(Harry's Cosmeticology)*

	%
Mineral oil	18.0
Glyceryl stearate (SE)	15.0
Pure water	55.0
Glycerine	5.0
Cetyl alcohol	2.0
Spermaceti	5.0

Perfume and preservatives may be added if desired.

Floral or Herbal Buttermilk Cleansing Milk for Normal or Dry Skin

1 cup buttermilk
2 tablespoons flowers of elder, lime, camomile or other blossoms

For a richer cleansing milk, full cream milk may be used instead of buttermilk.

Heat all the ingredients in a double saucepan for 30 minutes. Do not boil. Leave to infuse for 2 hours and then strain.

Yoghurt Cleansing Milk for Oily Skin

	%
Natural yoghurt (not pasturised)	75.0
Lemon or orange juice	25.0

TONING LOTIONS

These are used to tone or freshen the skin after cleansing and to remove the residue of the cleanser.

Flower Waters

These usually contain flower extracts, pure water and a preservative. They are the mildest form of toning lotion. They are suitable for dry and sensitive skin.

Flower Water *(Harry's Cosmeticology)*

	%
Potassium alum	4.0
Glycerine	6.0
Single rose water	35.0
Orange flower water	35.0
Pure water	20.0

Other perfume and preservatives may be added if desired.

Flower Water for Dry Skin

	%
Single rose water	75.0
Witch hazel	25.0

Flower Water for Oily Skin

	%
Single rose water	50.0
Witch hazel	50.0

Skin Tonics

These are a little stronger than flower waters and often contain spirit. They may also contain camphor which will stimulate and close the pores. They are suitable for normal or combination skin.

Skin Tonic *(Harry's Cosmeticology)*

	%
Denatured ethanol	20.0
Pure water	72.0
Propylene glycol	5.0
Laneth-10 acetate	3.0

Perfume and preservatives may be added if desired.

Marigold Tonic for Dry Skin

	%
Marigold infusion	60.0
Single rose water	39.0
Tincture of benzoin	1.0

Marigold Tonic for Oily Skin

	%
Marigold infusion	65.0
Witch hazel	34.5
Tincture of benzoin	0.5

Astringents

These may include zinc sulphate and tannic acid as well as herbal compounds. They are suitable for oily or heavy, mature skin.

Astringent (*Harry's Cosmeticology*)

	%
Alcohol	10.0
Zinc sulphate	0.5
Citric acid	1.0
Sorbitol	6.0
Pure water	82.5

Perfume and preservatives may be added if desired.

Lavender Astringent

3 tablespoons lavender flowers
1 tablespoon powdered orris root
$\frac{1}{2}$ teaspoon lemon oil
7 fluid ounces wine vinegar

Seal together in a bottle and leave to blend for two weeks. Disturb occasionally. Filter before use.

Rosemary Astringent

5 tablespoons vodka
2 tablespoons witch hazel
1 teaspoon glycerine
$\frac{1}{4}$ teaspoon borax
10 drops rosemary oil

Allow to stand for one week in a sealed bottle. This should be applied to the skin and not drunk!

ANTISEPTICS

These come as a cream or a lotion. They are used to kill bacteria on the surface of the skin. There is a wide range of proprietary brands available.

MASKS

The main purpose of a mask is to cleanse the skin. Most masks are used to remove dead skin cells, soften comedones, and to absorb oil and grease from the skin surface. Some masks are rather astringent, some are used to stimulate the skin while others have a calming effect.

There are five basic types of mask: wax, rubber, earth/clay, vinyl resin and hydrocolloids.

True masks should possess the following properties:
They should be a smooth paste.
When drying, they should form a coating over the skin.
They should be easily removed from the face by peeling off or gently washing off with warm water.
They should produce a tightening feeling in the skin.
They should cleanse the skin.
They must be non-toxic.
They should not have an objectionable odour.

A mask should be spread all over the face and neck but avoiding the hairline, the eyes, the nostrils and mouth. It may also be spread over the *décolleté*.

All-purpose Mask (*Harry's Cosmeticology*)

	%
Kaolin	35.0
Bentonite	5.0
Cetyl alcohol	2.0
Sodium lauryl sulphate	0.1
Glycerine	10.0
Nipagin M	0.1
Pure water	47.8

Perfume may be added if desired.

Properties of Ingredients for Clay or Mineral Masks

Bentonite is useful as a basic ingredient in a mask as it absorbs water and forms a gel.

Borax is mildly astringent and is useful in cases of acne to stop irritation.

Calamine has a soothing effect. It is useful in cases of inflammation or irritated skin.

Fullers earth has a deep cleansing effect as it absorbs oils quickly.

Kaolin has a deep cleansing effect and increases the blood flow to the area.

Magnesium carbonate (light) is a good base ingredient. It is astringent and helps to tone the skin.

Sulphur dissolves dead skin cells on the surface of the skin. It is very useful in cases of acne because of its drying effect on the skin.

Titanium oxide is soothing with healing properties. It has an absorbing effect on oily skin.

Zinc oxide is mildly astringent but also has a soothing effect. It helps to dry an oily skin.

Glycerine absorbs moisture from the atmosphere so keeping the mask soft.

Orange flower or **rose water** both have a soft toning effect.

Witch hazel has a drying effect and is a stimulating astringent.

Masks for Dry Skin

Mask for Dry Skin

1 part light kaolin
1 part magnesium carbonate
Glycerine
Rose water

Mix to a smooth paste. Leave to dry on the skin for 10–15 minutes.

Mask for Dry Congested Skin

Kaolin
Glycerine
Rose water

Mix to a smooth paste. Leave on the skin for 10–15 minutes.

Mask for Blanching or Softening Dry Skin

Fuller's earth
Glycerine
Rose water

Mix to a smooth paste. Leave on the skin for 10–15 minutes.

Mask for Sensitive Skin

1 part kaolin
2 parts magnesium carbonate
2 parts calamine
Rose water

Mix to a smooth paste. Remove from the skin before it dries out, approximately 6–8 minutes.

Masks for Oily Skin

Mask for Oily Skin

Fuller's earth
Witch hazel

Mix to a smooth paste. Leave on the skin for 15–20 minutes

Mask for Oily Congested Skin

Kaolin
Witch hazel

Mix to a smooth paste. Leave on the skin for 15 minutes.

Mask for Oily Skin Types with Acne

Sulphur
Witch hazel

Mix to a smooth paste. Leave to dry on the skin.

Masks for Normal Skin

Mask for Normal Combination Skin

1 part light kaolin
1 part Fuller's earth
Rose water

Mix to a smooth paste. Leave on the skin for 15 minutes.

Mask for Congested Normal Skin

Kaolin
Orange flower water

Mix to a smooth paste. Leave on the skin for 10 minutes.

Mask for Blanching and Softening Normal Skin

Fuller's earth
Orange flower water

Mix to a smooth paste. Leave on the skin for 10 minutes.

Biological (Natural Produce) Masks

A number of fruits, vegetables and household ingredients can be used to make a simple but effective mask.

Almond refreshes a dry or dehydrated skin and can be used to stimulate. It may be used as ground almonds in a paste or as almond oil.

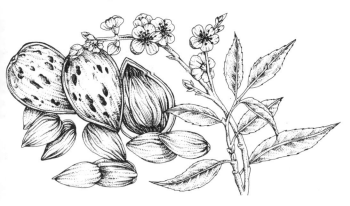

Avocado is very gentle on the skin. It contains a number of vitamins and minerals. It is very useful for cases of dry or sensitive skin.

Bananas are high in potassium. They also contain calcium, phosphates and vitamins. They are useful for dry and sensitive skin.

Cucumber has a very cooling effect and may safely be used on dry or sensitive skin. Cucumber slices make very good eye pads.

Eggs, both the yolk and the white albumen, may be used on normal or oily skin types to help remove comedones or other impurities. They are too drying for sensitive or dry skin.

Honey can be used to remove impurities and dead skin cells. It lightens skin and has a hydrating effect. It should not be used on young or sensitive skin.

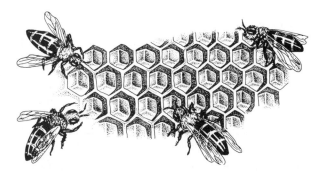

Orange or **lemon** juices are both very stimulating. They help to dry an oily skin and have a softening effect.

Olive oil is very good for nourishing dry or mature skin.

Oatmeal is used to remove comedones and to stimulate the skin, especially if it tends to be oily.

Papaya is very nourishing for a dry skin.

Potato helps to reduce 'puffy' tissues. Thin slices may be used as eye pads.

Yoghurt makes a very good base for masks.

Two or three of the above ingredients mixed together make a very effective mask. Remove gently with warm water.

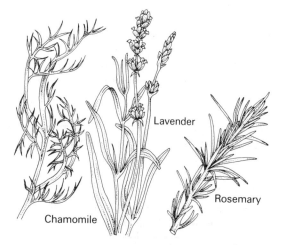

Masks for Dry/Sensitive Skins

Mask for Sensitive Skin

Oatmeal
Yoghurt
Mix together to make a paste. Leave on the skin for 5–10 minutes.

Mask for Dry Skin

$\frac{1}{2}$ banana
Ground almonds
Olive oil

Mix together to make a paste. Leave on the skin for 5–10 minutes.

Mask for Congested Dry Skin

Bran
Olive oil
Honey

Mix to a paste. Leave on the skin for 5–10 minutes.

Mask for Normal Skin

> **Mask for Normal Skin**
> Oatmeal
> Juice of $\frac{1}{2}$ orange
> Mix together to make a paste. Leave on the skin for 10 minutes.

Masks and Facial Scrubs for Oily Skin

> **Mask for Oily Skin**
> Oatmeal
> Egg white
> Juice of $\frac{1}{2}$ lemon
> Mix to a paste. Leave on the skin for 10 minutes.

> **Facial Scrub for Oily or Congested Skin**
> Salt
> Olive oil
> Juice of $\frac{1}{2}$ lemon
> Rub very gently with the fingertips over the skin surface. Leave on for 5 minutes.

EMULSIONS

It is said that oil and water do not mix. This is quite true if there are no other ingredients. Even if they are vigorously shaken up, the oil globules float to the surface. If a substance called an *emulsifying agent* is added, this breaks up the oil into very small particles. The oil can then be mixed into the final substance without the molecules joining together to form a large globule once more. There are a number of substances which will act as emulsifying agents such as borax or sodium hydroxide.

There are two types of emulsion: *oil in water* emulsion and *water in oil* emulsion.

Oil in Water Emulsion

A small amount of oil is dispersed into a larger amount of water. This is known as the *disperse phase*. The water, into which the oil is dispersed, is called the *continuous phase*.

When oil in water emulsion is applied to the skin it does not normally feel greasy as the water adheres to the skin first. The oil is distributed over this. The water will evaporate leaving a thin film of oil over the skin. This is called the *residual film*.

Oil in water emulsion often has a cooling or soothing effect on the skin.

Water in Oil Emulsion

In this form of emulsion, there is a larger amount of oil and just a small amount of water to be dispersed into it.

These two forms of emulsion form the basis of all moisturisers, creams and milks etc.

MOISTURISERS

There are two basic reasons why the skin becomes dry: physiological changes and external factors. Physiological changes may be caused by the body's inability to produce sufficient fluid to replace that which is lost on the skin surface, or by the ageing process. External factors include a low humidity (which dries the atmosphere), and the influence of ultraviolet radiation.

A moisturiser is a simple film of emulsion which acts as a barrier to the skin's own moisture by holding the moisture in the epidermis. A moisturiser may include hydroxyethyl cellulose derivatives and glyceryl stearate.

A *humectant* is a substance which attracts moisture; in this case, to the skin. It often contains glycerol, ethylene glycol or sorbitol.

> **Moisturiser** *(Harry's Cosmeticology)*
>
> | | % |
> |---|---|
> | Stearic acid | 15.0 |
> | Potassium hydroxide | 0.7 |
> | Glycerine | 8.0 |
> | Pure water | 76.3 |
>
> Perfume or preservatives may be added if desired.

Moisturisers, both day or night creams, are difficult to make from 'natural' ingredients. A moisturiser needs to give the skin a matte finish so that make-up can be applied on top.

NIGHT CREAMS

These creams are similar to moisturisers but are designed to spread easily and to stay on the skin for several hours without rubbing off. They often contain mineral oil, lanolin and beeswax.

Night Cream *(Harry's Cosmeticology)*	%
Sorbitan sesquioleate	4.0
Ozokerite	8.0
Petrolatum	30.2
Mineral oil	10.0
Lanolin	12.0
Pure water	30.0
Lemon juice	6.0
Perfume or preservatives may be added if desired.	

HAND-CARE PRODUCTS

Manicures and pedicares are amongst the most frequently performed treatments.

Hand Creams or Lotions

These are usually oil in water emulsions. They spread easily over the skin but do not leave it oily or greasy. They often contain a protective agent such as allantoin, silicones or lanolin.

Hand Cream *(Harry's Cosmeticology)*	%
Stearic acid	15.0
Zinc stearate	5.0
Sorbitan stearate	1.5
Polysorbate-60	2.0
Sorbitol	6.0
Methylcellulose (4% aqueous)	25.0
Water	45.5
Perfume and preservatives may be added as required.	

Glycerine and Essential Oil Hand Cream	
Single rose or orange water	250 ml
Glycerine	70 ml
Cornflour	5 tablespoons
Essential oil of your choice	4 drops

Cuticle Creams and Removers

These are used to soften the cuticle so that it can easily be pushed back or even removed where it adheres to the nail. The ingredients are normally alkaline in character such as potassium hydroxide or trisodium phosphate. A humectant such as glycerine is often added.

Cuticle Remover *(Harry's Cosmeticology)*	%
Trisodium phosphate	8.0
Glycerine	12.0
Pure water	80.0
Perfume may be added if desired.	

Nail Enamel Removers

These contain solvents such as acetone, amylactate or ethyl acetate. They have a very drying effect on the skin. To counteract this, an *oil*, such as castor oil or an *ester*, such as butyl stearate, is added.

Oily Nail Enamel Remover *(Harry's Cosmeticology)*	%
Butyl stearate	5.0
Diethylene glycol monoethyl ether	10.0
Acetone	85.0

Nail Enamels

These contain solvents such as methyl acetate or acetone to give them fluidity, which quickly evaporate. Film formers such as nitrocellulose are used to help the enamel to spread easily. Resins are used to give a good lustre and to resist the action of detergents. Plasticisers are used to stop the enamel from flaking once it is dry. A variety of coloured pigments can be added to produce the final colour.

The pearly lustre used to be obtained by adding a crystalline substance such as guanine. This is made from the scales of various kinds of fish and is very expensive. Bismuth oxycholoride is a cheaper synthetic that is often now used instead.

Base Coat

Base coats often contain more resin than normal enamel to give a harder film. They are used for two reasons: to give a good adhesion to the nail, and to prevent any colour from the enamel staining the nail.

Top Coat

These are used to protect the coloured enamel from chipping and to improve the gloss effect. They contain a higher amount of nitrocellulose.

Nail Enamels *(Harry's Cosmeticology)*	Base coat %	Clear enamel %	Top coat %
Nitrocellulose	10.0	15.0	16.0
Santolite resin	10.0	7.5	4.0
Dibutyl phthalate	2.0	3.75	5.0
Butyl acetate	–	29.35	10.0
Ethyl acetate	34.0	–	10.0
Ethyl alcohol	5.0	6.4	10.0
Butyl alcohol	–	1.1	–
Toluene	39.0	36.9	45.0

PART C

Salon Management

Chapter 18

The Salon

When a therapist first qualifies there are many types of work available. Options may include working for someone else in a salon, at a health farm or even eventually on board a ship. The therapist may prefer to have a mobile practice, work at home or even open a new salon.

Before opening a new salon or even a room at home there a number of legal and administrative factors to be taken into consideration. The salon owner should have a good understanding of the following:

  Location and salon layout
  Equipment and products
  Legal requirements
  Advertising
  Accountancy
  Raising capital
  Buying or renting property
  Insurance
  Staff administration
  Sterilisation and hygiene
  First aid
  Electricity.

CHOOSING A LOCATION

Where a salon is sited is of great importance. The public tend to think that if a salon is situated in the fashionable area of a large town it must be good. This may or may not be true. However, overheads will be considerable and the clientèle may be seasonal.

A number of successful salons are sited in large department stores. They are very often franchised from a parent company. The store often generates a considerable amount of passing trade but it may have only a few regular clients. The hours worked are normally regulated by the store.

A number of hotels allow therapists to rent a small room where the hotel visitors may be treated, as well as 'outside' clientèle. Some hospitals may have a beauty room where a therapist can work. In some

instances therapists are even allowed onto the wards during certain hours. Quite a number of hairdressers have an arrangement whereby a therapist can rent a room or cubicle. The rent may be a stated amount each week or a percentage of the client fees. For those therapists who want to work for a short time there are beauty salons to be found in holiday camps. These have plenty of work in the holiday season but are often closed for the rest of the year.

To be successful the salon does not have to be large. However, it should have both regular clients as well as 'passing' trade. A salon may well be more successful if it is situated near a rail or bus route, if there are good facilities for parking a car, and if there are a few shops nearby so that clients can quickly buy supper on the way home. Even a pedestrian crossing nearby can make a difference. It should be within easy reach of a residential area or where a number of people work. If there are noxious smells from a chemical factory or the sound of car panel-beating nearby this would adversely affect the number of clients seeking treatment.

The therapist should consider what 'success' means in this context. It could be purely monetary, it could be the freedom to practice at whatever times one wants, or it could be just plain 'job satisfaction'.

Some very successful therapists have a room in their own home where they work. They choose the hours, how much they want to work, how much they want to charge and what treatments to offer. They are, however, subject to the same regulations as are the formal salons.

SALON LAYOUT

The layout of the salon or the single room is important. Some people employ an architect or a design planner to do this for them. Unfortunately these professional planners do not fully understand the minor, but very important details of what is essential for a working salon.

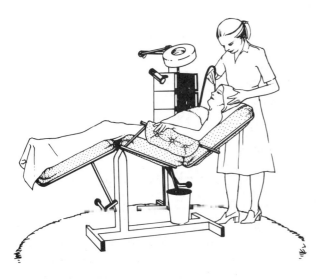

The reception desk should be tidy and uncluttered. The appointment book should be kept fully up-to-date and a note made for every treatment booked. Provision should be made for any money from cash transactions to be kept in a locked container. A receipt should be given each time money is accepted.

It is often a good idea to have a locked display cabinet showing all the items that you wish to sell. These may include a skincare range, make-up, nail polish, etc. Some salons sell a range of jewellery or even clothing such as leotards, T-shirts and swimwear.

Details of the fees charged for each treatment must be on display, as must the diplomas and certificates of the therapists working on the premises.

Changing Area

A place should be provided for clients to change their clothes and leave their possessions. Lockers should be provided if a number of people use the area. Cubicles should be large enough for people to turn around in and dress in comfort. Ideally, a stool and a table with a mirror should be provided so that make-up can be applied. Some women like never to be seen without it. A nice touch is to provide tissues, cotton-wool, cleansers, toners and a moisturiser for the client to use in the changing area. Toilet facilities should be nearby, with a wash basin, soap and clean towels handy.

Treatment Cubicles

The size of the premises often determines what sort of cubicle or area is available for performing the treatments. If just one small room of 3 m × 2.5 m (10ft × 8 ft) is available, you will need to work out carefully where to house the equipment. Is it to be kept in a cupboard until it is required or should it 'live' permanently on a trolley?

Reception

The first area of a salon that a new client sees is usually the reception area. Remember that the first impression is important. The area should have attractive wall coverings with perhaps a pretty picture or two. There should be two or three comfortable chairs, as some clients may bring a friend with them. If a client is only having a manicure this is sometimes performed in the reception area. New editions of a range of magazines should be available in case the client unfortunately has to wait a while.

Fresh flowers or pot plants will help to give a welcome. If smoking is to be allowed, the ashtrays must frequently be emptied and cleaned. There are still people who cannot go for any length of time without their 'fix of nicotine'. If herb teas, coffee or soft drinks are available, the empty cups must not be left lying around. This gives a very bad impression when people enter the salon. The area should be kept clean but have a friendly atmosphere.

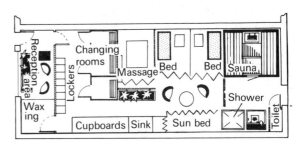

Salon layout

If the premises are large enough, there will be room for separate cubicles. Care must be used in deciding how to use them. Should one be used for each of the

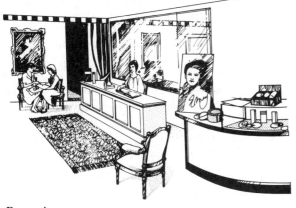

Reception area

main treatments such as electrolysis, waxing and facial massage, or should each of the treatments be performed in all of the cubicles? If this is the case, the equipment should be housed in one area and moved quietly when it is required.

Another point for consideration is the partitioning of cubicles. Solid walls give much more privacy. Curtains give more space, but everyone can hear what is being said.

Cubicles should be large enough to allow the therapist to walk all around the couch. There should be room for the various trolleys, magnifiers etc. Cleanliness should be evident. Therefore there should be a handbasin with hot and cold running water. Soap and clean hand towels or an air dryer should be available, though the latter can be rather noisy. A covered receptacle should be provided for rubbish.

Decor

This is a very personal matter. Do remember that in the salon a jazzy or psychadelic colour can excite the brain. A restful, pastel colour that is non-reflective will have a much more calming effect.

Lighting should be subdued with no direct overhead light. Few things are worse than opening one's eyes to stare directly into a lighted electric bulb. Wall lights are much kinder to clients' eyes. Natural daylight is fine for some treatments, but a sun-facing room at high noon in midsummer could be very hot and uncomfortable to work in. Rooms at the top of a building can often be very hot in summer and cold in winter if there is not a very good insulating system. A fan or air conditioning may be necessary, as well as an effective central heating system to maintain a comfortable temperature.

CHOICE OF EQUIPMENT AND PRODUCTS

The services that a salon can offer depends on what treatments the staff are capable of performing and on what equipment is available.

When starting a business there are a number of basic items that will be required. These include:
bins
bowls
client gowns
cotton-wool
couches

couch covers
forceps etc.
magnifyers
products
sterilisers
stools
tissues
towels
trolleys.

Do not be persuaded to have more equipment than you need, especially when first setting up a salon. Do not be persuaded to have impressive looking equipment which costs far more than a similar, but simpler, version. A more expensive version of a particular machine can always be obtained later when the equipment and treatment has been evaluated and proved profitable.

There is a very wide selection of equipment available. When setting up a salon, choose the equipment that is going to be used most. A machine will not pay for itself if it is only used once a week. Choose the treatments that the largest number of clients will want or need, and select this equipment. Further treatments and equipment can always be added later.

There is a bewildering array of products available for the therapist to buy and use. Some are very expensively packaged while others are much more simple. Large, well-known companies spend a lot of money on advertising. It does not mean that the products are the best available. Remember that the cost of advertising is always passed on to the consumer. Often the smaller manufacturer will have a product which is comparable or even better. The cost will usually be a fraction of the larger companies' product.

The therapist rarely has sufficient knowledge to distinguish between the good and the poor product. You will have to rely on what the manufacturer says, and may often be blinded by scientific jargon. The best way is to be guided by personal recommendation and through trial and error.

A number of manufacturers and agents have a minimum purchase value for their orders, which can often be several hundred pounds. The smaller companies usually have smaller amounts or even no restrictions. Most companies expect payment for the goods a month after they have been dispatched. Many only allow a fortnight and some expect payment before goods are sent.

It is very important to buy sufficient stock for use in the salon and for resale. There may be difficulty in getting products quickly if you run out, especially

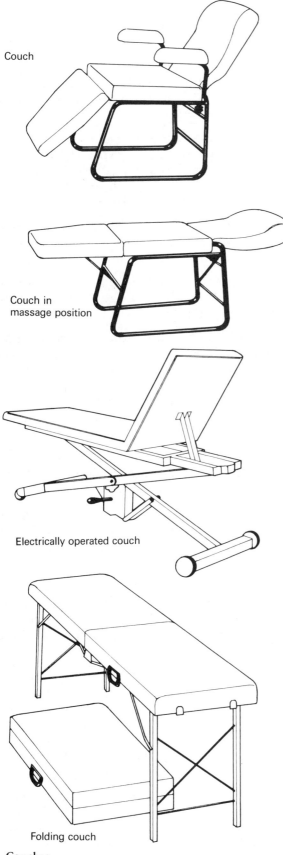

Couch

Couch in massage position

Electrically operated couch

Folding couch

Couches

during a holiday period. However, do not over-order products. Some products have a short shelf life and may deteriorate. Keep unused stock in a cool and preferably dark place.

Keep a card to record each product that you buy. Note the date, the size, the number of units and their wholesale and retail cost. This will help to build up a pattern of how frequently you need to replace any particular product in the future.

When buying new stock, it should always be placed behind the old stock. This way the old stock is always sold or used before the new, thus ensuring that only a fresh supply is used. If new stock is placed in front of the existing stock, the old stock may deteriorate and have to be wasted.

Retail products should have an individual price ticket so that the purchaser knows just how much is to be paid. Retailing can be a very profitable source of income. A number of salons pay a commission to therapists selling products. Selling products to clients can really be quite simple when giving them a treatment. Explain the benefits of the different products to the client and also how to use them. Each time the client returns, make a point of asking her if she is running out of anything.

Try to 'sell' the client the next treatment before they leave the salon. A client is more likely to come if they already have a treatment booked than if they have to phone for an appointment and risk their favourite therapist being booked already.

LEGAL REQUIREMENTS

One cannot just choose a location for a salon and say 'I will open a salon here'. There will be certain Local Government rules and regulations. If there is already a salon in the vicinity they could object to you opening near them.

Change of Usage

If the premises is not already a beauty salon, permission for a change of usage must be obtained. For example, if a small village has only one grocery shop and you wish to change this building into a beauty salon, the local residents could appeal to the Council as they would lose this local amenity. You would then be refused permission for a change of usage for that property.

Having obtained a property there is still a tangle of legal and licensing requirements before you can open as a salon.

Planning Permission

It may not always be possible to change the character of the property. The Local Council may stop you changing the external appearance of the property, such as enlarging windows or even adding awnings outside the windows. If the building is 'listed' as an old building, you could even be prohibited from changing the interior.

The Local Authority will not issue a licence unless the salon complies with a number of local regulations. These will differ from area to area. There are also a number of Government regulations.

Building Permission

Before starting any alteration of a structural nature, the Local Authority must give their permission. They will insist that the materials used are fire and weather resistant.

Very often the local Fire Prevention Officer will check on the fabric of the building. The width of the doorways and stairs will be checked. All the doors must be fireproofed and have automatic closure. The Local Authority may also wish to examine the ventilation and heating arrangements.

The Local Authority may wish to examine the washing and toilet facilities and to ascertain how you plan to dispose of waste matter or refuse. They will also be very strict about sterilisation.

A number of British Acts of Parliament cover the setting up and running of a business. Details of these can be obtained from the Department of Trade and Industry. Other countries have their own equivalent rulings.

The British law states that a minimum standard for cleanliness, safety and fire precautions are to be followed by those people working in a salon.

The law specifies how many fire exits there should be. This may depend on how many people work on the premises at a time. If the building has three or more floors, a second staircase or fire escape will be required. At all times the stairs and exits must be free of all forms of obstruction, such as boxes or ladders etc. The doors and exits must be clearly marked and must be able to be unlocked easily from the inside at any time.

Handrails must be provided on all stairways. Floor coverings should be held firmly in place and give a good foothold.

The law also lays down certain standards of hygiene. Sterilisers must be in a good state of repair and must be used. No one will benefit from having them on show as *objets d'art*.

Disposable items such as electrolysis needles should be placed in a sharps box. When this is full it has to be sealed and handed in to a hospital or health centre for proper disposal by burning. It should not just be placed in with the normal refuse.

Rubbish and waste materials should not be allowed to collect in stair wells or passages but put out for regular collection.

Instruments must be cleansed and sterilised each time they are used. Clean towels and couch linen should be used for each client.

The law also states that there must be adequate washing and toilet facilities with running hot and cold water, soap and clean towels for the staff and for clients. If there are more than five members of staff, separate washing and toilet facilities must be provided for both sexes. If there are more than ten members of staff, separate facilities must be provided for the clients.

The staff should have a separate room where they can relax and take their meal breaks.

The law stipulates that the minimum temperature of the workplace shall be 16 °C (60.8 °F) after the first hour of normal work. The temperature should not rise above 24 °C (75 °F).

The law states that there shall be an effective ventilation system in every room where the therapist will be working. There should be a minimum of 11.3 cubic metres (400 cubic feet) of space for each member of staff while working.

The law states that adequate lighting shall be provided. This may be natural or artificial. Equipment and fittings must be kept in a good state of repair. Basins and toilets must not be chipped but kept clean and hygienic. Chairs, tables, trolleys etc. must not remain broken because they can easily cause damage. All floor coverings must be secure.

All electrical equipment must be safe to use. Leads should not be frayed or allowed to trail across passages or walkways. Plugs and sockets must be correctly fitted. Any electrical faults should be repaired immediately. All electrical apparatus must be examined and tested by a qualified electrical engineer at least every six months. If the equipment is in constant use it should be checked more frequently.

Clean protective clothing such as overalls should always be worn when dealing with a client. However these should not be worn outside the environs of the salon.

The law also states that fire-fighting equipment must be provided and readily available. Fire drill should be held so that all staff know what to do in an emergency.

A first-aid box should be readily available and fully stocked.

The law lays down when a salon may not open. The Local Council rulings may vary from district to district but in general, shops and salons must close by 8.00 p.m. each night. They are allowed one late night (until 9.00 p.m.) per week. In holiday areas, the Local Council can alter closing hours for up to four months of the year. Some Councils permit late shopping at festivals or at Christmas time.

Shops or salons must have one half-day closing at 1.00 p.m. each week. This may be overcome by staff working split shifts or by having part-time staff. Normally salons do not open on a Sunday, though this is becoming more prevalent, especially in non-Christian districts.

The law states that goods or products should not be used or sold if they are hazardous to health. All goods must be suitable for the purpose for which they are sold. This means that if a client asks for a product that will perform an exfoliation and she is sold a normal cleansing milk, she may have cause for complaint.

When goods are sold that are not up to the standard or quality for which they were intended, then the seller is liable. Goods must be fit for their normal use.

No false information or claim may be given about goods, products or treatments. Goods and services must be described accurately. It is illegal to use a clause such as 'No refunds given' as this excludes the client's legal rights.

The size of the container must not be misleading, i.e. a very large container having a very small amount of the product inside it. Nor should the shape of the container be misleading.

Any ingredients listed should not deliberately set out to mislead the public. The purpose of the product must be stated. Also the method of use. Where a price reduction is indicated during a sale, the goods must have been sold at the original price in those premises for not less than 28 days.

No false or misleading claims for any treatments should be made in any advertisement or brochure or given verbally.

A number of Local Councils issue a licence to salons upon an annual inspection being carried out. The cost varies from £20–£150 depending on the area. It will cover most treatments except electrolysis and ear piercing, which require a separate licence. The inspection is usually carried out by an official from the Public Health Department.

ADVERTISING

There are a number of ways of advertising one's services as a therapist or salon. The most obvious one is to place an advertisement in a local paper. Sometimes it is possible to persuade the editor to mention you in an article on beauty. This may often be linked to a page of similar advertisements. An advertisement in a national glossy magazine is much more expensive. Remember that when advertising, the claims must be valid in every respect.

There are other ways of gaining the interest of the public. The name of the salon should itself cause interest. A special feature should be made of the windows so that the public want to see what you have to offer.

Advertisements giving special offers or a price reduction on certain treatments will help to get a salon noticed, especially if there is a different offer made each month.

A talk or demonstration at local Womens' Guilds or even schools will stimulate interest, as will coffee or wine and cheese evenings.

Some therapists, when working on their own, find that a leaflet put through the letterboxes of all the houses in the district will bring in clients.

It is not considered good professional business to place cards in the windows of such places as sweet shops or tobacconists. However it may be possible to leave cards at a local hairdressers, florists or good dress shop or outfitters and to ask them to hand them to any interested customers.

Local professional people such as doctors and chiropodists may send their patients to you if you can prove your worth to them.

FORMING A COMPANY

For a full listing of requisite business terminology, see Appendix B: Banking Terminology (page 200); Appendix C: Bookkeeping Terminology (pages 201–2); and Appendix D: Technical Terminology on Payment of Goods (page 203).

One difficulty that people find when starting a new salon is deciding what to charge for the different treatments. Fees are usually very much higher in the centre of large cities like London than in the suburbs or smaller cities. Fees will be less still in country areas.

A number of factors should be taken into account when setting the fees for treatments. They include:
 the time the treatment takes to perform
 cost of staff (including receptionist)
 cost of products used, laundry etc.
 cost of equipment, (rental costs or depreciation)
 property, rent or mortgage
 local taxes, VAT, corporation tax etc.
 electricity, lighting, heating, water
 telephone, postage
 advertising
 printing
 profit margin.

When a therapist is first setting up a salon she must decide if she is going to be: a *sole trader* (owner), a *partnership* or a *registered company*.

Sole Trader

This is usually a small business where there is one person who makes all the decisions, usually does all the work and keeps all the profits. They also have all the problems. They will be responsible for any staff, treatments, finances etc. If they get into financial trouble, their personal property as well as the salon can be seized to pay any debts.

A Partnership

In this situation, two or more people act as joint owners. One or more may actually work in the salon while others merely invest money in the venture. Like the sole trader, they raise the capital to set up the salon and are jointly responsible for any decisions, though only one person may have overall responsibility for the day-to-day running of the salon. They are also jointly responsible for any debts. If any member wishes to leave the partnership, the other partners usually agree to buy that share of the business.

A solicitor should be employed to draw up an agreement. This will show how much work (if any) each of the partners is responsible for. Partners do not necessarily own the business in equal proportions. The agreement will also show how the profits (or debts) should be shared.

A Registered Company

This can be: a *public limited* company, a *limited* company or an *unlimited* company.

A Public Limited Company

For this there must be a share capital of at least £50,000. The shares are usually held by a number of people who act as investors. They do not necessarily work for the company. A board of directors will decide the policy of the company and employ staff to manage and work in the business.

A Limited Company

This form of company must have at least two shareholders. They are only liable for debts of the company to the value of the shares that they hold.

An Unlimited Company

This is much more like a sole trader or partnership in that the shareholders are not covered for the amount of the debt should the company go bankrupt.

A registered company must have a document called a *memorandum* which gives details of the company. For all British companies this must be lodged at Companies House in London. An *unlimited* company is not necessarily a *registered* company.

Another legal document called an *article* states the rules for managing the company. It must include:
 the type of shares, i.e. voting or non-voting
 the number and value of shares
 how shares may be transferred
 rules for company meetings
 appointment and number of directors
 duties of directors
 members rights on voting and dividends
 procedures for accounting.

A register must be kept of the names of the members and directors, any financial interests of the directors and minutes of any meetings. Annual returns of the financial state of the company together with an auditor's and a director's report must be sent to the Registrar of Companies each year.

RAISING CAPITAL

Before starting any business it is necessary to know how much money will be required, both as capital expenditure and as working capital. A number of factors must be taken into consideration. For **capital expenditure** they include:

The premises: mortgage or rent, rating or local taxes.
Furnishings and fixtures: carpets, curtains, furniture, toilets, basins etc.
Decorating: cubicle dividers, lighting.
Equipment: bought or hired.
Products: for salon use or retail.
Advertising: in magazines, local papers, reduced cost of treatments, demonstrations.
Printing and stationery: brochures, cards, note paper, receipts.
Telephone: for salon use, payphone for client use.
Postage.
Legal fees.
Accounts fees.
Staff salaries.
Incidentals: books for accounting, cleaning items, laundry, magazines, books, flowers, coffee, soft drinks etc.

The **working capital** must also be estimated. This is the money that is required to meet all the expenses of running the salon until it is making a profit and can pay for itself. This must also include the interest to be paid on any loan as well as the agreed amount of the loan itself.

Besides working out how much money will be needed you will need to know whether it is to be borrowed all at once or in instalments. You will also need to know how long the money is to be borrowed for, and how and when it is to be repaid.

The next thing is to decide where to borrow the money from. There are several courses available. They include:

Family and Friends

If a therapist is going to start up a salon by working on her own, family or friends may be in a position to loan or donate money for this venture. The interest will generally be less this way.

Bank

Bank managers are normally quite reasonable people. The business of a bank is to lend money. The bank manager will want to see realistic details of how the money is to be spent and a forecast of how you expect the salon to proceed financially. Normally the borrower is required to offer some form of security. You could also be asked to put 50 per cent of your own money into the business.

Money can be borrowed for varying periods of time.

Loans

Long-term Loans

These can be arranged for between ten and twenty years. The interest to be paid will be the normal bank interest rate. For larger sums of money the bank will insist that the borrower is covered by a life assurance policy.

Short-term Loans

These can be from one to five years. They are a separate agreement with the bank, and would not be included in a personal current account. They should not exceed £1500 and are subject to the Consumer Credit Act (1974) which also covers hire purchase, credit and conditional sales.

Finance Houses

These are an alternative to the banks but their interest rates are usually higher.

A Bank Overdraft

This is money that may be borrowed on a current account. The interest is paid only on the money outstanding. However, the overdraft can be called in by the bank at any time. It is probably better to use this form of borrowing for working capital rather than for buying equipment.

Building Societies

These will normally loan money for the purchase of property or other large expenditure but not as working capital.

Hire Purchase

This can be used to buy any large piece of equipment. Payment is made usually to a finance house, of a specified amount for an agreed period of time and due at monthly intervals. Interest will have to be paid as this is a form of loan. The equipment remains the property of the hire purchase company until the total sum of money is paid.

Credit Sales

In this case, the equipment belongs to the purchaser from the beginning of the loan. The money, plus the interest, is repaid at an agreed rate over a stated period of time.

Hire Contract

This is a facility for renting equipment. A rental fee is paid monthly or quarterly and may be terminated by giving notice at an agreed period of time. The equipment never becomes the property of the salon. In most instances, the leasing company will carry out any repairs. This is a very useful method of hiring very expensive equipment.

PREMISES – BUY OR RENT?

Having worked out what the working capital, plus most of the capital expenditure will be, you must now decide whether to buy or rent property. This must, of course, depend on the present owners of the property.

Buying a Property

Freehold property means that the property and the land, if any, surrounding it and under it is owned outright.

Leasehold property means that the leaseholder buys and then owns the property for as long as the original lease was granted. Unless this lease is extended, at the end of the leasing time the land and any building on it revert back to the owner of the land. The lease-holder pays the landowner a nominal amount of ground rent each year.

Renting Property

An agreed amount of money is paid to the property owner at regular intervals. A lease agreement states how much is to be paid and how frequently; how often the rent will be reviewed; who is to be responsible for repairs, both inside and outside; and also for any decorating.

When either buying or renting a property it is considered essential to employ the services of a solicitor. They will deal with such things as land searches and all the small print in a contract.

INSURANCE

Insurance acts as a measure of financial protection for a stated risk in such instances as accident, damage by fire or flood, loss of earnings etc.

A *policy* is a contract made between an insurance company and an individual or a company (salon) known as the *insured party*. The party agrees to pay the insurance company a specific amount of money each year, called a *premium*. The greater the risk, the higher the premium. In return, should a risk occur, the insurance company agrees to pay the insured party a *lump sum* of money to replace property or goods damaged or loss of earnings etc.

A *proposal form* gives details of what risks are to be covered. It states how much each risk costs to insure and what the lump sum and replacement money would be. It gives details of when the premium is due and any special conditions issued in connection with the premium.

Insurance cover means having an insurance policy for a specific risk, e.g. a car. Insurance may be taken out for various risks. These include: *fire*, *flood* and *theft*. Very often these three risks are considered together, though in some instances they may be separate.

Fire may cover just a fire in a piece of equipment or the whole salon burning down. Smoke and fire alarms should be fitted and tested frequently. Fire-fighting equipment should be readily available.

Flood may involve just a soaked carpet or three feet of sea water in the salon ruining floors, walls and equipment.

Theft usually refers only to goods stolen following a break-in. It is very difficult to get an insurance company to agree to goods or equipment that 'walks out of the door'. The policy should include the theft of clients' personal effects though it is much easier to ensure that these are placed in a locker. Insurance companies normally require proof that the premises are secure, with door and window locks. A burglar alarm would also reduce the premium cost. Any cash kept overnight should be held in a secure safe.

When the contents of a salon are insured this may be at a 'depreciating value' in which case the premium will be quite low. Alternatively, the contents can be insured at a 'new replacement value', where the money paid will cover the cost of a new piece of equipment of the same or similar type. Very often insurance companies do not pay out the money until the new equipment has been purchased.

Plate glass and *mirror glass* may be insured separately. General policies do not often cover them.

A *loss of profit* policy may be taken out. If there is a flood or fire it may be several months before the salon is earning money again. If the salon owner has an accident and is unable to work for some time, money will be paid for this period. An extension of this could be for staff being attacked in the course of their work. This might be when carrying money to the bank or by an intruder breaking into the salon.

Car insurance: if a private car that is used to travel to and from work is also used to visit clients or to carry stock, the insurance company should be notified that it is also being used for business purposes. Failure to do so could leave the policy holder without cover and liable to pay any costs incurred in the case of an accident.

A *life assurance* or *endowment* policy states that when a person loses the ability to earn money due to accident or even death, their family should not suffer financially. The insurance company will pay a lump sum to the insured party or their relatives.

Employers Liability Insurance Act 1969. This is a compulsory insurance for any business either employing staff or for premises where members of the public may enter. It places certain responsibilities on the salon. It covers claims from clients in respect of an accident in the salon or negligence by the staff. It also covers claims from staff for any accident or negligence occurring in the course of their work and during their working day. The salon must, of course, ensure that safety standards are maintained by all members of staff at all times. Any accident or breach of safety must be fully recorded as soon as possible after the event.

STAFF ADMINISTRATION

Employment

When staff are to be employed, certain ideas and terms of work have to be agreed. At an interview the potential employer should give as many details about the job as possible. The interviewee should be able to ask a number of wide-ranging questions.

The Interview

The employer or salon manager should give a description of the work involved, i.e. whether the interviewee would be expected to perform electrical treatments as well as facial massage or manicure. Any possibility of special training in new techniques, or being sent on a course should be mentioned.

Very often an interviewee is expected to demonstrate an ability to perform different treatments at an interview.

A number of points should be discussed at the interview. They should include:

1 How much time is given to cleaning machines and trolleys between clients. Who is responsible for cleaning the salon each day. Is this done in the morning or the evening?
2 Who actually owns the salon. How they can be contacted outside the salon.
3 What the working week consists of: the number of hours a day, a week. Whether this involves split shifts, evening work, and working every Saturday. Whether it includes working on a Sunday. What provisions are made for meals or coffee breaks?
4 How many other people work at the salon. Who is responsible for making the bookings, taking the money. Are particular people responsible for performing special treatments?
5 Amount of salary. Whether commissions are paid on treatments and on sales of products. Is the salary still paid if clients do not turn up or there is a slack period? Total of contributions to be deducted. When the salary is paid: monthly or weekly; and how: by cheque or cash. Is overtime paid? Is there a starting salary? How long does this remain unchanged? Are there annual increases in salary?
6 Holiday arrangements. The length of holiday allowed each year. Whether this has to be taken all at once or when the salon wishes. Is the salon closed on bank holidays? Are the staff paid for these? Whether salary is paid for days off taken for emergencies. Is 'sick pay' given if longer periods need to be taken? Is the job held if an employee is away for even longer periods? Maternity leave. Pension scheme.
7 Will the work always be at the salon site or would the interviewee be expected to work at other branches?
8 Who is liable if equipment is damaged or products or money is missing during the working day?
9 Whether there is a procedure for grievances. Who would arbitrate? Are there any restrictions on Trade Union membership? What redundancy money would be paid?
10 Terms of notice: length required from either side prior to the termination of the job.
11 Whether there would be any restraint on the interviewee from working at a nearby salon on leaving this job. Many salons have a 'restraint' clause on former employees working nearby, e.g. within half a mile in a large town or two miles in a country area.

12 In some instances it should be made clear as to who provides the overalls, equipment and products.

13 The date that the job becomes available. The date the interviewee would be able to commence work.

14 Original references should be shown to the potential employer, who may wish to take details so as to seek confirmation later. Interviewees should note that the name of a referee should never be given unless they have first been asked if they are willing to give a reference.

15 Contract of work: is this a written or an oral one? Either type of contract is legally binding on both the employer and the employee. If there is a written contract the interviewee should read this carefully. If any point is not clear, it should be questioned. If a clause is not acceptable, negotiate or try to have it removed before the contract is signed. No document should be signed by either side until all the points are fully understood and agreed.

16 If no written contract is made, notes should be made as soon as possible for the conditions of work. A verbal contract is still legally binding.

17 Once a contract is agreed there are both rights and duties for the employer and the employee (see below). A contract comes into effect as soon as the job is offered and accepted and both parties agree to the conditions of the contract. An employee can, by law, demand a written contract showing details of the conditions of employment within the first thirteen weeks of employment.

Employer Duties

To implement the terms of employment agreed in the contract. To make sure that employees are aware of what is required of them.

To give or arrange training where new techniques are required. To negotiate changes in working practices and schedules as required. To try to arrange a good working schedule, i.e. neither too many nor too few clients.

To provide equipment and premises that are both safe and suitable for the work required.

To ensure that staff are qualified to perform specialist treatments on the public.

To pay the agreed salary for work performed according to the contract. To pay the agreed commission. To pay the Government taxes such as Income Tax and National Health contributions and to keep a record of such deductions and salaries. To pay the Public Indemnity insurance in case of an accident to a client or member of staff.

To provide suitable first aid should it be required.

To treat staff with proper courtesy and respect. To allow no prejudice or discrimination on grounds of sex, colour, creed, race or age.

Employee Duties

To implement the terms of the employment agreed in the contract. To be ready and willing to work on clients. To take all reasonable care when working on clients, e.g. to carry out a 'patch test' when necessary. To carry out all reasonable requests with regard to work within the agreed terms of the contract. To negotiate changes in the working practice and schedules.

To ensure reasonable care and to account for all equipment and products used in treatments. To account for any money taken as fees. To indemnify the employer for any loss as agreed in the contract.

To work for only the employer during the working day. Not to disclose any professional trade secrets used at the salon.

To treat all staff with courtesy and respect. Not to exercise any prejudice or discrimination in respect of staff or clients.

Termination of Employment

A salon may not unfairly dismiss a member of staff. An employee may demand (by law) a written reason giving details of why the employment is being withdrawn.

On leaving a salon the employee may request a reference. This request may not be refused. It must be an accurate statement without derogatory remarks. Employers, therefore, tend to make generalised statements. Rather than mention that an employee came in late four or five times a week in an inebriated state, the reference might state that the employee arrived in a convivial state on a number of mornings each week.

Any employee who has been working for less than two years should give or receive one week's notice. Between two and twelve years, the notice should extend by one week for each year's service. If the employee has worked for over twelve years the period of notice should be twelve weeks. Very often an appropriate amount of money may be negotiated in lieu of the employee working out the notice time.

Redundancy

In some instances a job may 'disappear'. The business may close or go bankrupt. There may not be sufficient work for all the staff. This can often happen where there is seasonal work and the particular skills of that person are no longer required.

Redundancy payment can be claimed by full-time employees with more than two years employment. If staff are put on short-time or are laid off for four weeks or longer they may be considered to be redundant.

Reasons for Fair Dismissal

1 The work no longer exists, therefore the employee is redundant.
2 The employee would be breaking the law if they continued to perform the work.
3 The employee is found to be unqualified to perform the work.
4 The employee is not able to perform the work because of ill-health.
5 The employee's performance of the work is so bad that it is not being performed adequately or safely.
6 The employee's conduct is unsatisfactory.

Misconduct is a frequent cause for dismissal. It can include: persistent lateness or leaving early; taking too long over lunch breaks etc.; persistent careless-ness and misuse of stock; repeated damage to equip-ment; rudeness to clients and other members of staff; general untidiness and poor performance of work.

If misconduct occurs the employee should receive a formal verbal warning, stressing that failure to improve could result in dismissal. If the misconduct continues, a written warning should follow. Again the consequences should be stressed. If the misconduct occurs yet again the employee can face suspension without pay for a stated period of time or even dismissed.

Reasons for Instant Dismissal

This is a very grave situation indeed. It can only be carried out for gross misconduct where either there is a witness or it can be proved beyond all doubt.

Gross misconduct can include: theft of equipment, stock, client's effects or property belonging to other members of staff; stealing money from the till; deliberate damage to the equipment, stock, salon etc.; malpractice or injury to clients or other members of staff.

Industrial Tribunal

If an employee feels that they have been unfairly dismissed they may apply to an Industrial Tribunal. This is a board formed from professional people and specialists in the same field. There may also be lawyers, Trade Union representatives and members of ACAS. They will hear the case as put by both sides. They will then discuss and arbitrate the case. They may decide that the salon was right to dismiss the employee. If they feel that the dismissal was unfair they may either have the employee re-instated at the salon or specify an amount of compensation to be paid to the employee.

STERILISATION AND HYGIENE

A knowledge of sterilisation and hygiene is of great importance to the therapist. Bacteria breed in an unhygienic atmosphere. They can cause infection of a local or general nature. Therefore cleanliness must be observed.

Bacteria can be carried in the air as spores. Food poisoning is caused by certain bacteria being ingested. Bacteria in pus from boils and wounds can be transmitted by direct contact with it. Viruses, like the common cold, are transported through the air as a droplet infection. Viral diseases such as AIDS or hepatitis can be transmitted during pregnancy to the baby, through infected blood transfusions, sexually, or through contact between infected material and cut or grazed skin. Sterilisation and hygienic procedures must be carried out in order to prevent the spread of any infection.

Bacteria are capable of breeding outside a host. Some are capable of quite rapid growth. Many are able to multiply even after being frozen. Some bacteria require carbon dioxide for growth, others need oxygen. They all require a suitable acidity (pH) of 5–9, but usually between 7.2 and 7.6. The best temperature for bacterial growth is 37 °C/98.4 °F (which is also body temperature), though they can grow in conditions below freezing and up to 80 °C/ 176 °F.

Spores

These are not yet bacteria but in the right atmosphere they can germinate into a single bacterium. Bacterial spores are particularly difficult to kill as they are highly resistant. They need a much higher temperature or strong chemical before they can be made safe.

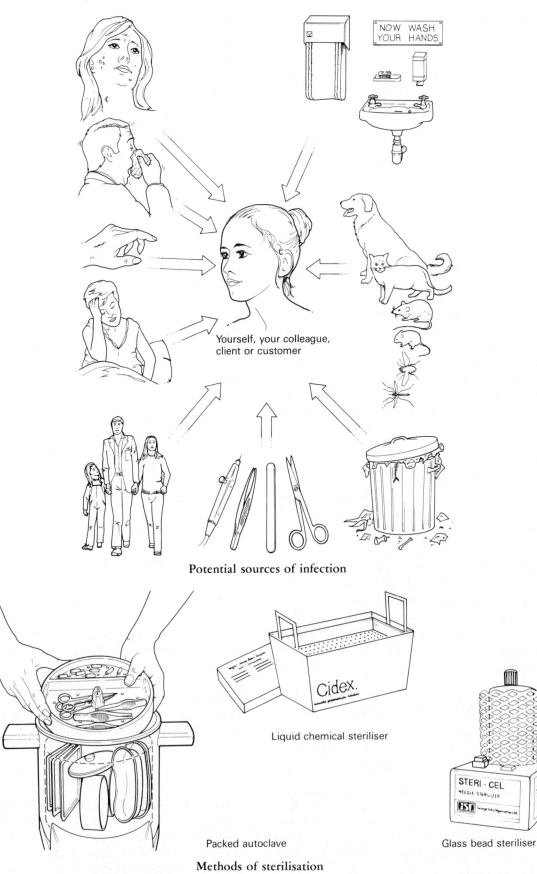

Potential sources of infection

Liquid chemical steriliser

Packed autoclave

Glass bead steriliser

Methods of sterilisation

Viruses

Viruses are inactive outside of a host. However, the herpes simplex virus can be transmitted by contact and the common cold can be caught by being near to someone sneezing.

Fungi

Fungal infection is often reduced where there are bacteria. When these are supressed by the use of a broad-based antibiotic, fungal activity may be increased. The fungus *Candida albicans* causes the condition known as *thrush*. This can affect the inside of the mouth, the vagina and in some cases even the skin and nails. *Trichophyton interdigitale* is the cause of *tinea pedis* (athletes foot). This can be transmitted from one infected person to another through the use of the same towel.

A therapist owes a duty to her clients, her colleagues and herself to protect them from all sorts of infection.

Killing Bacteria

Bacteria and other organisms may be killed by the use of different methods such as the use of:
    disinfectant
    antiseptic
    bactericides
    biocide, sporicide, fungicide or virucide
    sterilisation.

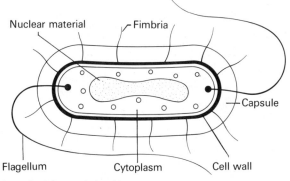

A typical bacterial cell

Disinfectant

The word disinfectant is normally used for a solution that is applied to an inanimate object such as a couch or floor. It will reduce the number of bacteria on a surface though it will not usually kill bacterial spores. Aqueous solutions should not be used on electrical equipment in case water seeps into the components. This would subsequently cause damage to the equipment.

Antiseptic

This term is defined as 'against' (anti) and 'putrefaction' (septic). An antiseptic is used to destroy or inhibit bacteria and other micro-organisms. It is made as a solution and is usually applied to the skin.

Bactericide

This is a chemical agent which will kill bacteria but not bacterial spores, fungi or viruses.

Biocide, Sporicide, Fungicide and Virucide

These, as their names imply, are chemical agents which kill all forms of 'life' in spores, fungi and viruses. They are frequently used to soak instruments which may come in contact with these micro-organisms.

STERILISATION

The term *sterilisation* means 'the killing of all bacteria, spores and viruses.' Sterilisation may be achieved by the use of:
    heat, both dry and steam
    radiation
    chemical liquid.

Before any item is sterilised it is very important that it is thoroughly cleaned.

Dry Heat Sterilisation

Hot Air Ovens

In order to be at all effective this type of steriliser needs to be used at a temperature of above 150 °C (302 °F). Some sophisticated models even reach 280 °C (536 °F). The lower the temperature, the longer the instruments need to be in the steriliser. For example:
instruments heated to
    160 °C (320 °F) require 45 minutes
    170 °C (338 °F) require 18 minutes
    180 °C (356 °F) require $7\frac{1}{2}$ minutes
    190 °C (374 °F) require $1\frac{1}{2}$ minutes.

Items placed in a heat steriliser must be capable of withstanding the high temperature. Plastics, ordinary glass, cloth or brushes are not suitable for this form of sterilisation.

Glass Bead Sterilisers

These consist of a metal cylinder containing very small glass beads (see page 141). Different models heat up to 190–300 °C (374–572 °F). The sterilisation times range from 30–60 minutes. Because of their size they are only suitable for the very smallest articles such as forceps, comedone extractors or electrolysis needles.

Steam Heat Under Pressure

Equipment used for this type of sterilising is called an *autoclave* (see page 142). It works on the same principle as a pressure cooker. Steam is produced from a reservoir of water and is contained under pressure. Sterilisation time at 134 °C (273 °F) is approximately 12 minutes.

Bowls and receivers should be placed on their side and not upside down so that the steam touches the entire surface.

Radiation

Some items, notably electrolysis needles, are supplied already sterilised. Each needle is pre-packed and then bombarded by radio-isotopes such as colbalt-60.

Sterilisation using ultraviolet may be used for certain items. Ultraviolet will only sterilise where the rays actually fall. Therefore it may only be used for items having a solid surface such as forceps. They need to be turned over during the sterilisation period. It is not suitable for items such as brushes or sponges, as the rays cannot penetrate them.

Liquid Chemical Steriliser

This consists of a 'plastic' container which has a perforated tray inside it (see page 182). The sterilising fluid is composed of chemical compounds called *aldehydes*. They have proved to be very effective for short-term sterilisation. After 14–28 days, depending on the manufacturer's method of production, the molecules come together to form polymers. These render the solution ineffective. The most widely used chemical is glutaraldehyde as a 2 per cent aqueous solution.

Great care must be taken to see that the solution is changed at the recommended time, after the stated number of days. A note of the date for changing should be placed in a prominent place.

All instruments should be thoroughly cleaned and dried before being placed in the solution. Any water will reduce its potency.

To be fully sterilised, instruments should be left in the solution for 30 minutes.

Sterilising fluid can severely damage the skin. Instruments should be removed from the solution with a pair of long forceps, placed in a receptacle and rinsed well to remove any traces of solution. The instruments should then be dried and stored ready for use. Some people even take the precaution of wearing rubber gloves when handling the solution. If any solution gets onto the skin it should *immediately* be washed off. If any solution gets into the eyes, they should *immediately* be washed with copious clean water and then medical attention sought.

Any instruments that have a damaged or worn surface should be discarded as they may retain a residue of solution.

Waste Disposal

All waste matter such as cotton-wool, tissues or dressings must be disposed of with the greatest care. Ideally, it should be placed in a plastic bag, tied up and then placed inside a second bag. All electrolysis needles that are not re-sterilised should be placed in a sharps box for incineration.

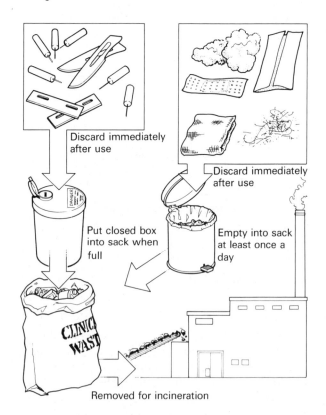

Discard immediately after use

Discard immediately after use

Put closed box into sack when full

Empty into sack at least once a day

CLINICAL WASTE

Removed for incineration

It is of the utmost importance that hygienic methods are used, and are seen to be used.

FIRST AID

Accidents should not happen, but they do, even in the best run salons. Clients can become unwell, they may have had an accident on the way or something can happen in the salon. All therapists should therefore know something about first aid.

If anyone requires first aid or is involved in an accident, however minor, details should be fully recorded in a book specially kept for this purpose.

Every therapist should know where the first-aid box or container is kept. Someone should be responsible for seeing that it is kept fully stocked.

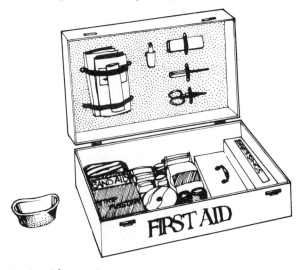

It should contain:
  a thermometer
  headache or pain 'killers'
  antacid tablets or liquid
  individually wrapped plasters in assorted sizes
  sterile gauze coverings in various sizes
  cotton bandages in assorted sizes
  crepe bandages in different widths
  surgical adhesive tape in assorted widths
  sterile eye pads
  triangular bandages
  tissues and cotton-wool
  safety pins
  scissors
  eye bath
  forceps (for removing splinters etc.)
  cold compress
  antiseptic lotion
  burn cream or gel
  paraffin gauze dressings
  antiseptic medical wipes
  petroleum jelly
  information cards giving the name, telephone number and address of the local doctor.

The following are conditions which could unfortunately occur in a salon.

Asthmatic Attack

This may be occupational, allergic, hereditary or of nervous origin. It is caused by the muscles of the air passages going into spasm. The passages may also become blocked with mucous. The warning signs include noisy, wheezing breathing, and often a difficulty in exhaling. The complexion may be pale with beads of sweat on the forehead.

Action
1 Sit the patient up, leaning forward with their arms resting on a table or on the back of a chair.
2 Loosen the clothing.
3 Give the patient as much fresh air as possible while still keeping them warm.
4 Give the patient their own medication if it is available.
5 Gently rub the patient's back. This can often give relief.
6 If the attack is severe, seek medical assistance.

Bleeding

Minor external bleeding, abrasions and cuts.

A number of people are affected by the sight of blood, however little it may be. In most small cuts, the bleeding will stop spontaneously by the formation of bloodclots.

Action
1 Abrasions should be washed clean with warm water and a mild antiseptic solution. Care must be taken to remove any grit or other foreign matter. If it cannot all be removed, especially on the face, the patient should be seen by a doctor.
2 Cover the area with a pad of dry, sterile gauze.
3 Small cuts should have a pressure pad applied to them for about ten minutes. Apply a sterile dressing.
4 If there is a foreign object such as a sliver of glass in the wound, the pressure should be applied along the side of the cut. A light sterile dressing should be applied and medical assistance sought to remove the foreign body.

Severe External Bleeding

When there is severe bleeding the patient may go into a state of shock. The skin may become pale and feel cold and moist to the touch. There may be profuse sweating. Breathing may become shallow and yawning and sighing may occur. The patient may feel faint. The pulse rate may increase but feel weak.

Action

1 If the patient is in danger of fainting, lay them down and raise the feet.
2 Apply a sterile dressing to the area.
3 If the wound is in a leg or arm raise the affected limb so that the blood runs away from the area.
4 Send for an ambulance or medical help. It is often a good idea to send two people for help in two different directions just in case one of them does not get through on the telephone.

Nose Bleeding

This could be caused by a severe injury, in which case send for an ambulance. Most nose bleeding, however, is caused by a rupture of the small capillaries inside the nose.

Action

1 Sit the patient up, with the head forward.
2 Ask the patient to breathe through the mouth.
3 Pinch the nostrils firmly together. Hold for about ten minutes or until the bleeding stops.
4 Ice may be applied to the area. An ice cube may also be given to the patient to suck.
5 If the liquid from the nose is a clear, watery fluid, it could possibly be cerebrospinal fluid. Seek medical help immediately.

Bruises (Contusions)

This occurs when blood has escaped into the dermis, subcutis or underlying tissue. There may be soreness, swelling and discolouration.

Action

1 Check that there are no other injuries such as laceration or, more seriously, a fracture or internal bleeding.
2 Apply firm pressure to the area with a cold compress or an ice pack or place the limb in cold running water. Cooling the area has the effect of slowing down the bleeding.
3 If the bruising is extensive, the pain severe, or there is difficulty in moving, the patient should see a doctor.

Burns and Scalds

Burns are caused by dry heat. Scalds are caused by moist heat. Burns may be classified as superficial, intermediate and deep, according to the depth of the burn. A superficial burn affects the epidermis only. There will be redness, swelling and tenderness. An intermediate burn affects the dermis. There will be redness, swelling and blisters, and the burn will be painful. Deep burns can affect the subcutis and underlying muscles. The skin may be pale, waxy or even charred. There will not be a great deal of pain as the underlying nerves will have been damaged.

If a quarter of the skin's surface is burnt the condition is considered to be serious, as plasma will escape from the burn and therefore the blood volume decreases.

Action

1 For superficial or intermediate burns, immerse the burn in cold water or place under running cold water for ten minutes.
2 Apply a sterile dressing if necessary.
3 Do not attempt to break a blister.
4 If the area of the burn is larger than 2.5 cm ($\frac{1}{8}$ inch) and includes more than just the surface of the skin, medical attention should be sought.
5 If the burn is severe, seek medical attention immediately.

Electrical Burns

If a burn is obtained from a piece of electrical equipment, switch off the electrical current, preferably at the mains or at the meter.

Action

1 If the person is unconscious or still in contact with the equipment, *do not touch* either the equipment or the patient until the current has been switched off at the mains (do this quickly). If this is not possible, stand on a rubber mat, or even a pile of newspaper which will act as an insulator. Use a *wooden* broom handle or wooden chair to push the electrical cable and equipment away from the patient.
2 Place the patient in the recovery position.
3 Send for an ambulance and treat the patient for shock.

Cramp

This is a painful muscular spasm. It can be caused by poor muscle coordination, by muscles being chilled (as when swimming), or by loss of body salts through excess sweating, vomiting or diarrhoea.

Action

In the hand: Straighten the fingers and press down onto a hard surface. Massage the afflicted muscles while they are being stretched.
In the foot: Stand on the ball of the foot and flex upwards. Massage the afflicted muslces.
In the calf: Flex the foot upwards and stretch the calf muscles while massaging them.
In the thighs: If possible sit on the floor. Stretch the muscles at the back of the leg by pushing the knee down. Massage the afflicted muscles.

Diabetes

Most people who suffer from diabetes know how to cope with their disorder. However two conditions needing action can arise: a *diabetic coma* and an *insulin coma*.

Diabetic Coma

This condition can arise because there is a reduction in the level of sugar in the blood. It can be caused by exercise burning up the blood sugar, by eating too little sugar in the diet or by taking too much insulin.

The appearance of the skin will be pale and sweaty with a clammy feeling. The pulse will be rapid and weak. The breathing will be shallow and rapid. The patient may become confused, sometimes resembling drunkenness. There will be *no* odour on the breath. The patient will first become faint and then rapidly deteriorate into a coma.

Action

If the patient is *conscious*, give three or four teaspoons of sugar or honey, chocolate, or a sweet drink. Make sure that the sweeteners are not synthetic.
If the patient is *unconscious*, place in the recovery position and send for an ambulance immediately.

Insulin Coma

This condition arises when there is too much sugar in the blood. Usually the patient will be aware of the condition and treat themselves with insulin.

The skin will appear flushed and dry. The breathing will be deep, rather like sighing. The breath will smell strongly of acetone (or pear drops). Unconsciousness will occur more slowly than in a diabetic coma.

If the patient becomes unconscious, place in the recovery position and send for an ambulance immediately.

Epileptic Fit

This is caused by a disturbance in the cerebral cortex. There are two forms: *petit mal* and *grand mal*.

Petit Mal

In petit mal there is a momentary confusion but not a loss of consciousness.

Grand Mal

In grand mal the patient may have a warning a few seconds before an attack.

The patient will become unconscious. There will be convulsive movements. The muscles become rigid and then relaxed. The teeth may be clenched together. Occasionally the tongue may be bitten. There may be a loss of bladder or bowel control. When consciousness returns, the patient may be drowsy and confused.

An epileptic fit can be quite an unpleasant experience to observe, though there is nothing to be afraid of.

Action

1 Protect the patient from hurting themselves by removing furniture near them. If possible place a pillow under the head.
2 Loosen clothing if possible.
3 Do not move the patient from the area unless they are in danger, such as from falling off a couch.
4 Do not restrain the movements.
5 Do not try to put anything into the mouth to hold the tongue.
6 When the convulsions cease, place the patient in the recovery position.
7 Stay with the patient until they have recovered.
8 An ambulance need only be called if there is a series of fits, if the patient is unconscious for longer than fifteen minutes or if the patient injures themselves.

Fainting

This is caused by a temporary reduction in the blood supply to the brain. It is often the result of sudden pain, a sudden fright or emotional stimulation, a drop in the blood sugar level caused by missed meals or dieting, or standing still for too long at a time.

Before they faint, the patient will become very pale, sweat will appear on the face, neck and hands, and the skin will be cold and clammy.

Action

If a person *feels faint*, sit them down and put the head down between their knees. Loosen any tight clothing.

If the patient actually *loses consciousness*:
1 Raise the legs above the level of the head by putting them on a chair or even holding them up.
2 Loosen any tight clothing.
3 Make sure that the patient has plenty of fresh air.
4 Apply smelling salts to the nose.
5 When the patient is fully conscious give them sips of cold water. Do not give any alcohol.

Objects in the Eye

It is quite common to get objects such as an eyelash or grit under the eyelids.

Action

1 Tell the patient not to rub their eye. This will only make it worse.
2 Sit the patient down facing a light.
3 Tilt the head backwards.
4 Gently lift the upper eyelid or draw the lower lid down to find the foreign object.
5 Lift it out with the corner of a clean handkerchief or rolled tissue.
6 Tell the patient to blow their nose. Quite often this will dislodge the object.

Chemical Burns

Tilt the head sideways and wash out the eye with water directly from a tap or use a jug. Continue to wash out for at least ten minutes. Gently cover the eye and get the patient to a Casualty Department as soon as possible.

Objects Impaled in the Eye

Do not attempt to remove the object. Cover the eye with an eye pad, taking care not to apply any pressure to the object. Get the patient to a Casualty Department as quickly as possible.

Sprains

This is an injury to a joint when the ligament holding two bones together is wrenched. The joint will be tender and discoloured. There will be swelling over the area. Moving the joint will cause pain. In some cases it can sometimes be mistaken for a fracture.

Action

If possible, apply a cold compress within half an hour of the injury. Then apply a bandage firmly around the joint so as to immobilise and rest it.

Strains

This is when a muscle is overstretched or ruptured. There will be a sudden, sharp pain in the muscle followed by stiffness and swelling. The area may become discoloured and develop cramp.

Action

Treat by applying a cold compress to the area for half an hour. Then apply a firm, but not tight, bandage. Rest the limb.

Strokes

A stroke is a loss of blood to one side of the brain. It may cause weakness or paralysis to one side of the body or even unconsciousness.

Action

If the patient is *conscious*:
1 Support the head and shoulders on cushions.
2 Turn the head to one side to allow saliva to drain from the mouth.
3 Call an ambulance immediately.
4 Loosen clothing.
5 Do not give anything to drink.

If the patient is *unconscious*, place them in the recovery position.

Heart Attacks

This is caused by lack of blood to the heart muscles. The patient will have severe pain in the chest, often spreading down the left arm and even to the right arm. The patient may become breathless and sweat profusely.

Action

If the patient is *conscious*:
1 Support them in a semi-recumbent position. Place a pillow under the knees. Loosen any clothing.
2 Do not give anything to drink.
3 Send for an ambulance.
4 While waiting, do not let the patient make any unnecessary movement because this will place extra strain on the heart.

If the patient is *unconscious*, place them in the recovery position and send for an ambulance.

Artificial Respiration

If the patient has stopped breathing the brain will become starved of oxygen and they will die within minutes. Artificial respiration must be given.

Action

1 Make sure that the airway is clear.
2 Remove any debris from the mouth.
3 Tilt the head well back so that the tongue does not obstruct the airway.
4 Wipe a handkerchief or a piece of material over the patient's mouth.
5 Pinch their nose with the thumb and forefinger.
6 Place your mouth over the open mouth of the patient. Breathe in through your nose. Breathe out through your mouth. Continue doing this for two or three breaths at a normal rate of breathing.
7 Check to see if the patient's chest is moving. Repeat until an ambulance arrives or until the patient resumes breathing.

Recovery Position

If an unconscious person is left lying on their back they could choke on any saliva, blood or vomit.

Action

1 Lay the patient straight on the floor. Cross the far ankle over the one nearest to you. Place the far arm across the body and the near arm straight, under the body.
2 Pull the patient's body over towards you.
3 Tilt the chin to prevent the tongue from obstructing the airway.
4 Bend the arm and leg nearest to you to stop the patient rolling onto their back.
5 Wait with the patient until help arrives.

HOW ELECTRICITY WORKS

Electricity is generally taken for granted. It is not always treated with the respect it deserves. This is a pity because electricity can be highly dangerous.

There are three basic units of electricity:

Voltage can be thought of as the force of the electricity. The domestic voltage of the UK is 240. It differs in other countries.
Amperage indicates the rate at which the electricity flows.
Wattage indicates the amount of electrical power. It is a measurement of the rate at which a piece of equipment uses electricity.

An electric light bulb on average uses 40–100 watts. An electric fire will use 3000 watts (3 kilowatts).

$$\frac{\text{watts}}{\text{volts}} = \text{amperes}$$

$$\frac{3000 \text{ watts}}{240 \text{ volts}} = 13 \text{ amperes}$$

This formula shows how to determine the correct fuse or size of electric cable for a piece of equipment of a known wattage.

Fuse

It is very important to know how many amperes a particular piece of equipment requires so that the correct fuse can be placed in the plug. A fuse is a piece of wire of a known resistance. It acts as a safety device to prevent overloading of the cable and subsequent damage to the equipment, or even harm to the therapist or the client.

There are three types of fuse: *wire* fuse, *cartridge* fuse and *circuit* breaker.

It is important that a cartridge fuse of the correct amperage is put into a plug. Do not use a higher amperage fuse than is required for that piece of equipment.

Sometimes a fuse will 'blow'. If this happens repeatedly it may indicate that there is a serious fault either in the equipment or in the cable.

Wire Fuse

Before attempting to look at a mains fuse the electricity must be switched off at the mains. It is a good idea to have the fuse holders marked to indicate which circuit it controls. It is also useful to have a few spare fuse holders already wired with the correct fuse wire, e.g. 5, 10 or 15 amperes.

Having found which fuse has blown, loosen the screws that hold the broken wire. Remove the old wire. Cut a length of new fuse wire of the correct amperage. Wrap the ends of the wire around the screws in a clockwise direction so that when the screws are tightened they will not dislodge the wire. Replace the fuse in the holder. Replace the fusebox cover. Switch the power back on.

Cartridge Fuse

In a cartridge fuse, the fuse wire is encased in a cartridge. There is no way that just the wire can be replaced; the whole cartridge has to be replaced. The plug fuse is a form of cartridge fuse.

Circuit Breaker

A circuit breaker is really a switch which automatically shuts off the circuit if it becomes overloaded. It will cut off all electricity to the cable if it itself becomes damaged. For example, there is a circuit breaker in electric lawn mowers, which may run across their own leads. Without a circuit breaker anyone who picked up a cut lead would be electrocuted.

Wiring Up a Plug

When wiring up a plug, care must be taken to ensure that the correct colour wire is connected to the corresponding pin:

Brown wire to the *live* pin on the *right*.
Blue wire to the *neutral* pin on the *left*.
Green/yellow wire to the *earth* pin at the *top*.

Quite often the plug will be marked. It may have a diagram showing which wire should be attached to which pin.

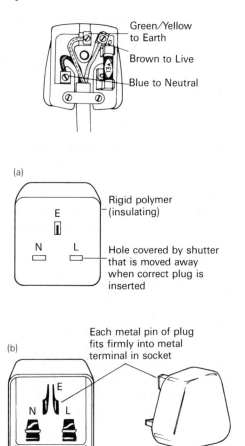

The live and the neutral wires complete an electrical circuit with the equipment. The earth wire drains excess electricity harmlessly away from the equipment.

In the plug, screws holding the wires should be firmly tightened so that the wire cannot be pulled out.

Faulty Equipment

If a piece of equipment does not function correctly, switch off the electricity at the wall. Pull the plug out by hand, not by pulling on the cable. Check the wiring and the fuse inside the plug. Never attempt to repair equipment while it is still plugged in.

Most equipment manufacturers will rescind any guarantee for the equipment if it has been touched by anyone other than one of their own engineers. Obtain full details of where to send equipment if it should ever need attention.

How to Avoid Damage to Equipment

Keep all equipment clean and free of dust or oils. This is one of the main causes of failure.

Do not let any fluid or oil seep into the inside of the equipment.

Avoid having trailing leads. These may be a hazard because people can trip over them. Trolleys will not easily run over trailing leads: they may become tangled in the leads and so pull on the plug. If a trailing lead has to be used, make sure that it can easily be seen. A verbal warning should be given to anyone going near it.

If an adaptor is to be used make sure that you are not using too much equipment, otherwise this will cause overloading. Unless it is absolutely unavoidable, it is much safer not to use an adaptor, but to have a number of sockets around the room.

Safety

Never remove a plug by pulling on the wire. Always switch off at the socket and then carefully remove the plug by holding the plug itself.

Switch off all the electricity at the socket when it is not being used. All plugs should be removed from the sockets at the end of the day or when not in use. Frequently check the wiring inside the plug.

Ensure that any equipment used directly on a client is properly earthed. Buy equipment from a reputable source. Remember that some equipment may look good on the outside but be totally unsafe inside.

All equipment should be frequently checked by a qualified electrical engineer.

Chapter 19

The Client

Although men do visit beauty salons, this occurs relatively rarely. The following chapter assumes that in most cases your client will be a woman, although the advice given may also apply to a male client.

RECEPTION

At all times the comfort and care of the client is paramount. She must be made to feel welcome as soon as she enters the salon. A client should not be left to wait in the reception area without someone attending to her. If a short wait is unavoidable, she should be shown where to sit, offered a magazine or something to read and told how long the delay is likely to be. If it is longer than five or ten minutes she should perhaps be offered something to drink such as a fruit drink or herb tea.

A woman usually comes to a salon because she feels that she has a problem and needs help. She may have unwanted hair. She may suffer from tension. She may be overweight. It is not enough merely to perform electrolysis, a massage or a faradic treatment. The client should be helped to understand her problem and how it can be treated. She will need understanding and even sympathy. For her unwanted hair she should be told a little about how the hair grows and how electrolysis can help her. She should also be told that it can be painful. A good electrologist, however, will be able to minimise this discomfort both by her technique and by her sympathetic attitude.

Gaining Confidence

A relaxing massage or facial treatment can help to alleviate tension. By asking the right questions and carefully listening to the answers, a good therapist can often pinpoint the cause of the tension and so may help the client to avoid, or at least lessen it in the future.

With the overweight client, the therapist must first win the client's cooperation and then try to find out when and why she first became overweight. The client should then be persuaded to go on a calorie reduced diet. Only after that is it time to discuss what the specific treatment should be.

The therapist must build up the confidence of the client. Where possible the client should always be seen by the same therapist at each appointment so as to maintain continuity of treatment. If the client sees a new person each time, she may lose her confidence and not bother to continue with her treatment.

Where possible the client should enjoy her treatment and look forward to her next visit. She must have confidence in her therapist and respect for her knowledge, realising that the treatment she is receiving is the correct one for her. She must feel that she is receiving value for money, both in time and treatment.

The client must never be embarrassed by word or action. For example, the therapist should never tell a client that she is 'fat', but could suggest that she may perhaps be a little 'overweight'. The client should never feel that someone can see her having a treatment through a window. Curtains or blinds should be used where there is a danger of the room being overlooked.

The therapist will become used to seeing people unclothed. The client however may feel a sense of modesty in undressing in front of another person. Her privacy must be observed when she is disrobing. A cubicle or screened area should be provided. A gown or towels must be provided to cover her. The client must be clearly instructed on how much clothing she should remove for the treatment.

The client must always be helped on to the couch, covered up and made as comfortable as possible. A loosely rolled towel placed under the small of the back can sometimes relieve back tension.

At all times the client must be kept warm. In hot weather the atmosphere should be cooled as much as possible without chilling the client.

RECORD CARDS

It is an essential part of the therapist's work to keep a record of her clients, their treatments and their progress.

Name	Address
Sex Age	
Doctor's Name	
Telephone No.	Telephone No. Home/Work
Medical History	

Date	Treatment Received	Other relevant details

The details on the card should include name, address, phone number (daytime number if working, as well as home number), age, sex, reason for the visit and any general observations.

It should be noted whether the client suffers from such conditions as diabetes, epilepsy, cardiac or upper respiratory problems. The skin type and condition should be noted. If a manicure or pedicare is to be performed, the state of the hands and feet should be

HEALTH & BEAUTY CLINIC		
Name Mrs. P. Smith	**Address** 21 Bantland Rd, Felixport FX1 2dB	**Tel.** 19674
Skin diagnosis Dehydrated skin. Tendency to dilated capillaries. Sensitive to lanolin. Loss of skin tone in neck area.		

Date	Treatment record	Special care & cosmetic sales
19.9.79	Continental facial. Lip wax	HOME CARE ADVISED - cleansing preparations
26.9.79	Continental facial. Eye brow shape	- toner (tissue firmer)
3.10.79	Warm oil mask therapy	- night cream
10.10.79	"	- under makeup nutrient base
24.10.79	Continental facial / Indirect H/F	
31.10.79	" Lash + brow tint	MAKEUP PREPARATIONS - tinted foundations
	Makeup	- powder/cream eye shadows
12.11.79	Facial with muscle toning. Lip wax	- non-allergic lipstick; tawny pink
		- mascara; dark brown

noted. Recent surgery and any other medical data, including allergies, should also be noted. The name and address of the client's doctor should also be on the record card.

After each visit, the date and the treatment given should be recorded. Adverse details from the previous treatment should also be recorded.

CONSULTATION

The consultation should take place the first time that the client meets the therapist. It is important to make a good impression on the prospective client and to create an air of confidence. Professionalism is the keynote. The therapist should be able to discuss and to advise on what she feels is the best treatment for that client. It may not be quite what the client envisaged, but if she is persuaded that this is the treatment that she requires, she will usually agree to having it. At no time must the client be persuaded to have a treatment that she does not need.

The client must be left in no doubt as to the full cost of the treatment or series of treatments. She should be informed if there are any extras. She should never be presented with a bill for the treatment plus a host of hidden extras. This will only embarrass her. There must be complete honesty on the part of the therapist. The therapist should never recommend an expensive treatment when a cheaper treatment would serve the condition just as well.

During the consultation the client should have details of the treatment fully explained to her and have the opportunity to ask questions. At the end of the consultation the client should feel confidence in the therapist and look forward to her treatment.

In some cases it is advisable for the treatment to follow on after the consultation. Occasionally the client will go home, and because she is unsure of the treatment, may change her mind and cancel. If she has had one treatment, and enjoyed it, she will usually return for others.

Chapter 20

The Therapist

It is possible to train almost anyone to become a therapist. It takes considerably more to train someone to be a good one. The therapist will have to learn how to observe people: how they sit, whether they are relaxed or tense, whether they have any skin problems, the conditions of their hands, whether they need electrolysis, and many other points.

The therapist needs to learn how to communicate with people. She needs to be able to help people to relax so that they can discuss their particular problem.

First impressions count. When the client meets the therapist for the first time it is her appearance and attitude that determines how well the treatment goes and whether that client will return for further treatments.

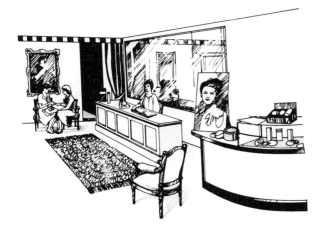

PERSONAL STANDARDS AND HYGIENE

The therapist should have a pleasant and cheerful manner. It is important to know when to chatter and when to keep quiet so that the client can relax. It helps to have an interest in several subjects so that the conversation will consist of more than just comments on the weather. Reading a daily paper or a magazine regularly will help to widen one's ability to discuss various topics.

The therapist's appearance must be clean and tidy. Some form of overall should be worn at all times. It need not necessarily be white. A pale pastel colour can look very smart without being too clinical. A touch of informality may help a nervous client to relax. Whatever the colour, the overall should be well-laundered, without any tears or lost buttons. A number of female therapists now wear white trousers. Overalls should not be too tight, otherwise stretching becomes difficult.

If the therapist is entitled to wear a badge from an examination board or a professional organisation, she should wear it with pride. It is a token of her qualification, a recognition of a standard. It sets her apart from those who are not formally trained. The therapist should not wear any conspicuous jewellery such as dangling earrings. A pair of small stud earrings may be worn. Chains, bracelets and rings should not be worn because they can catch on the client. They can collect oil and become very unhygienic. They may also cause problems when performing certain treatments, such as high-frequency treatment. For the same reason, watches should not be worn on the wrist, but be pinned to the overall or kept in a pocket. Any jewellery looks out of place and unprofessional.

The hair must be clean and worn off the face. If hair is allowed to fall about the face, it will look untidy, get in the eyes and the therapist will be continually pushing it back. Female therapists with longer hair could wear it plaited or in a pony tail.

The therapist's skin must be seen to be clean. Blemishes should be attended to and any stale make-up should be removed. If worn, make-up should be carefully and discreetly applied.

Clients can be frightened off if they feel that a therapist is too sophisticated. They may fear that she will be unapproachable. They may hesitate to ask the very question that is worrying them. The therapist should not be over-elaborate in her dress or over-bearing in her manner.

Oral hygiene is very important. A regular visit to a dentist is advised. Frequent use of toothpaste and mouthwash is most important. If one enjoys hot spicy foods extra care should be taken and an oral deodorant used. People who smoke must also take extra precautions because the smell of nicotine lingers on the breath and the hair and comes out through the skin and sweat.

It is essential to be particular about one's personal hygiene. The judicious use of soap and water and a deodorant will help to keep one's body fresh. If you wish to wear a perfume, or in the case of a man, an aftershave, it should not be overpowering. A light cologne would be sufficient.

The hands must be well manicured and the nails kept short. If they are long it is impossible to perform many treatments effectively. A nail digging into the skin during a facial treatment or massage is not a pleasant experience, nor is the rasp of rough skin. If nail enamel is worn, it must not be smudged or chipped. Hands must be thoroughly washed before and after every treatment and during it if necessary.

As the therapist is standing for most of the day, it is essential to wear comfortable shoes. It is a good idea to change them during the day. They must be kept clean and in a good state of repair.

The above points of personal standards and hygiene should be adhered to at all times. It is only a courtesy to one's clients to present a personal freshness to them. A therapist who is untidy or lazy about their personal appearance is likely to be untidy or lazy in their work.

ATTITUDE TO CLIENTS

A therapist must always maintain a professional attitude towards clients.

The client who is being treated deserves your undivided attention. Put thoughts of the previous client out of your mind and do not start to think of the next client until you have finished with the present one. Do not allow thoughts concerning your personal life to distract you: concentrate solely on the client.

Do not discuss a client's condition or personal life with anyone else. Anyone who gossips will soon lose her clientèle.

Be prepared to listen sympathetically to clients but do not become involved in their problems. Do not give direct personal advice unless you are a trained counsellor.

When clients consult you about a treatment, do not let them dictate which treatment they should have, nor how it should be carried out. You are the expert. Just because a certain treatment is right for Mrs X it does not mean that it is the correct one for Mrs Y. However, you must take into account the client's wishes.

Keep your problems to yourself. Clients may want to unburden their problems on to you but will not particularly wish to hear yours. The old Victorian adage of avoiding the topics of sex, politics and religion still make sense. This way one avoids disagreement with a client.

PROFESSIONAL ETHICS

A therapist's relationship with others in the same field as well as with members of other professional bodies is of great importance. Therapists should respect one another. If you cannot find anything good to say about another professional's work, it is better not to say anything. Because one therapist has been trained in a different way from oneself, it does not mean to say that either way is correct or incorrect. The methods are just different. Instead of disagreeing, it is much better to get together and exchange ideas.

When therapists work together in a salon they must present a united professional front to the clients. They must agree to carry out the same treatments in the same manner. The treatments should not be altered without consulting the person responsible for that treatment.

The therapist should not accept any clients for a treatment who are currently receiving the same treatment elsewhere, unless they have the permission of the other therapist. In other words, do not poach.

On leaving employment with a particular salon, do not try to entice clients away from your former employer, or go into business in the near neighbour-hood.

The therapist should strive to have a good under-standing with others in the 'beauty world'. If one has the chance to go to different exhibitions one should take them. One can always see new ideas that are worth trying and get to talk to other professional people.

If a therapist can gain the confidence of the local doctors, they are quite likely to recommend their patients to the salon. If a doctor does send a patient or a specific treatment the therapist must carry out that treatment as directed. A therapist must never attempt to treat a medical condition without a doctor's permission.

By the same token, a therapist may perform a pedicare, but any advanced foot treatment should be referred to a chiropodist. We do well not to tread on their toes!

When you accept a person as a client you must give them your full attention and the best treatment of which you are capable.

One should be prepared to accept a person as a client regardless of colour, creed or personal circumstance.

CONCLUSION

When you have completed your training and leave your school or college, you may find that your professional life is not as easy as you anticipated. Salons may not come up to your expected standards. Some may not be as clean as you would wish. In others, treatments may be performed with more haste than you would like. If you are working on your own, there may be a shortage of clients to begin with. Whatever happens, do not lower your own standards but try rather to raise the standards of others.

Whenever you can, seek to improve your knowledge in all aspects of your work. So much is happening in this profession that one should be continually adding to one's original knowledge, studying new techniques to see if they will work, discarding those that do not.

Be proud of your profession. May you have great success and personal satisfaction from it.

Chapter 21

Examination-type Questions

In each of the questions below, the question number corresponds to the chapter number in which the answers can be found.

1 a) State what is meant by the following:
      i) cephalic   iii) distal
      ii) posterior   iv) superficial.

2 a) Draw and label a diagram of a cell.
   b) With the aid of a diagram, describe the process of mitosis.
   c) Draw and label three types of simple epithelial cells and say where they are found.
   d) Draw and label three types of loose connective tissue and say where they are found.
   e) List the composition of bone.
   f) Draw and label a diagram of a muscle fibre.

3 a) Draw and label two diagrams showing all the layers of the skin and structures within them.
   b) Describe, in detail, the eight functions of the skin.
   c) Describe eight abnormalities or disorders affecting the skin.

4 a) Draw and label a diagram showing the bones of the skull.
   b) List, describe and give examples of the five classifications of bones.
   c) Name, describe and give examples of the three types of joints.
   d) Describe the two types of bone.

5 a) Name and describe the three types of muscle tissue.
   b) Name and describe six muscle shapes.
   c) Draw and label two diagrams showing at least twenty-four facial muscles.

   d) List, describe and give points of origin and insertion for the muscles of facial expression and mastication.

6 a) Draw and label a diagram showing the main parts of the brain.
   b) Describe how impulses are transmitted along a nerve pathway.
   c) List, giving the type and function, the cranial nerves that have an effect on the face and head.
   d) State what a motor point is and draw a diagram to show where twelve of them lie on the face and head.
   e) State the functions of the sympathetic nervous system.

7 a) Draw and label a diagram of the heart and state which way the blood flows through it.
   b) List, in order, the arteries supplying the face and head from the heart.
   c) State the composition of blood. Say how it differs from lymph.
   d) Describe how the lymphatic system functions.

8 a) Name, describe and state the position of all the endocrine glands.
   b) Give a definition of an endocrine gland.
   c) State the functions of five of the endocrine glands.

9 a) Draw and label a diagram to show the bones of the hand and wrist.
   b) Draw and label a diagram of a nail.
   c) Describe the three stages of hair growth.
   d) List the muscles of the lower arm and hand and say what action they have.

10 a) Describe how to perform a skin analysis.

b) Describe eight skin types.

c) Explain what is meant by the term 'allergy'.

d) Describe, in detail, how to cleanse the skin.

e) Explain how to perform exfoliation.

f) List the contra-indications to exfoliation.

11 a) Describe how to perform all the main movements of a facial massage.

b) Discuss the reasons for giving a facial massage.

12 a) Describe, in detail, how to perform an ultraviolet treatment.

b) List the contra-indications to an ultraviolet treatment.

c) Describe the routine that the client should follow prior to having an ultraviolet treatment.

d) State the reasons for giving an infra-red treatment.

e) List the contra-indications or precautions that should be observed when performing an infra-red treatment.

f) Describe, in detail, how to perform a facial steam treatment.

g) Describe one other method of warming the tissues.

13 a) List the reasons for performing high-frequency.

b) List the contra-indications to high-frequency.

c) State the differences between the two methods of performing high-frequency.

d) Explain the principles of the galvanic current.

e) List the contra-indications to galvanism.

f) Describe, in detail, how to perform ionto-phoresis.

g) Describe the four types of faradic surge patterns.

h) Explain the anticipated effects of faradism.

i) List the contra-indications to faradism.

j) Describe how to perform a vacuum suction treatment.

k) Give the reasons for performing vacuum suction.

14 a) Draw and label a diagram showing the bones of the foot and ankle.

b) List the blood vessels supplying the foot.

c) Explain how to perform a manicure.

d) Describe four types of nail shape.

e) Describe eight disorders affecting the nails.

f) Describe how to repair broken nails.

g) Explain how to perform one type of nail extension (sculptured nail).

h) Describe how to perform a foot and leg massage.

i) Describe one other nail and hand treatment.

j) Explain how and why hygiene and sterilisation techniques should be observed.

15 a) List the contra-indications to depilatory waxing.

b) Describe how to perform depilatory waxing.

c) State the after care required for depilatory waxing.

d) Explain how to shape the eyebrows.

16 a) With the aid of diagrams, show how to apply blusher for five different face shapes.

b) State how you might recognise an allergy to make-up.

c) Explain how to sterilise make-up brushes and other instruments that may be used in a make-up.

d) Explain how to tint eyelashes and eyebrows.

e) Explain how to determine the correct shape for eyebrows.

f) Describe how to apply strip lashes.

g) Describe how to bleach facial hair.

17 a) Explain the difference between a deodorant and an antiperspirant.

b) Explain the differences between flower water, skin tonic and astringent.

c) Explain the reasons for applying a mask.

d) List the ingredients that may be used in three different types of masks suitable for dry skin.

18 a) Discuss the legal aspects of setting up a new salon with regard to local licensing authorities.

b) Discuss the different ways that money may be obtained for acquiring a suitable property and equipment for a new salon.

c) Discuss at least ten points that should be dealt with at an interview for a job.

d) List the reasons for fair dismissal and for instant dismissal.

e) Discuss the importance of sterilisation.

f) Describe four methods of sterilisation.

g) List the items that should be contained in a first aid box.

h) State what action should be taken if the following conditions occur in a salon:
   i) fainting   iii) a heart attack.
   ii) a sprain

i) Explain how to wire up a three-pin plug.

j) Discuss the precautions that can be taken to avoid damage to electrical equipment.

19 a) Discuss the importance of keeping record cards.

b) List all the appropriate headings to be included on a record card.

c) Discuss carrying out a consultation with a new client.

20 a) Discuss the qualities that are required in a good therapist.

b) State what points should be considered to ensure a good code of Professional Ethics.

Appendix A:
British Standard 3456.102.27

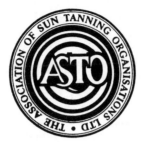

In the interests of safety, all sun tanning equipment should conform to the British UVA Standard. These should be at least 99% UVA because that is the safest way to tan. There are two types of equipment that conform to this Standard.

Low Pressure Equipment:
This equipment uses fluorescent tubes. They are usually 6ft long and commercial equipment has between 20 and 35 tubes set into a canopy and base. Some tubes emit less than 99% UVA. Make sure the equipment you buy conforms to the British UVA Standard. When you replace the lamps ask for written confirmation that your equipment will remain within the British UVA Standard with the new lamps.

High Pressure Equipment:
This equipment has lamps instead of fluorescent tubes and is very expensive. However, it gives out much more UVA so you can achieve a tan much more quickly than with the conventional type of sunbed. The bare lamps are very dangerous so the equipment is usually key-locked for safety. Thick 'bullet proof' glass ensures that only pure UVA penetrates through to the user. Always make sure the glass is properly fitted and not cracked.

If the amount of UVB coming from an appliance is more than 1% then according to the British Standard it should be labelled UVB. There are two types of UVB equipment:

Low Pressure Equipment:
Skin is highly sensitive to UVB and so medical science condemns it as being too dangerous to use for sun tanning. However, appliances which should be labelled UVB are often instead given names like 'high speed' or 'fast tanning'. The hazards of UVB exposure are well documented and your clients should not be using it. It is easy to identify as it causes the skin to go pink after only about 20 minutes.

Face Lamps:
Very old-fashioned equipment has an even higher level of UVB and causes burns in just a few minutes. This has been condemned by the Consumers Association as only fit for the rubbish heap. They say: 'Do not give it to a jumble sale, you are only passing on the problem to someone else.' So any lamp (or equipment sometimes called a solarium) which causes burns in a matter of minutes should never be used for sun tanning purposes. Whatever protection it may offer the skin from sunlight is of little consequence compared to the long term risks of exposure to this sort of radiation.

Appendix B: Banking Terminology

A **cheque** is given in place of money. It may be exchanged at a bank or similar business house for cash, providing there is sufficient money in the account on which it is drawn.

An **open cheque** is exchangeable for cash at a bank.

A **closed cheque** can only be paid into an account. It is therefore safer than an open cheque if it is lost.

A **cheque card** serves as a means of identification. It also guarantees the card holder's cheques up to a stated value, usually £50 or £100.

A **current account** is a 'spending' account. The account holder is given a cheque book, cheque card and a paying in book. Goods and services may be paid for by cheque, providing there is sufficient money held in the account or other arrangements are agreed with the bank. Money to be paid into the account is entered into the paying in book as well as onto the counterfoil. When a cheque is written, the counterfoil should also be filled in with the amount. Thus an accurate record on the account is kept.

A **deposit account** is a 'saving' account. Interest is paid on the money saved in the account. It cannot be used directly for paying out money as there is no cheque book.

A **cash dispenser** is used with a card to obtain cash up to the value of £200 at any time providing there is sufficient money in the account.

A **night safe** allows businesses to deposit money safely in the bank after bank closing hours. The holder uses a key to open a deposit door in the outside wall of the bank. The money is placed inside in a special container. This goes down a chute into a safe. The container may be retrieved, unopened, by bank staff the following day.

A **credit card** is an alternative method of paying, rather than by cash or cheque. A plastic card containing a code relating specifically to the card holder is placed into a small unit. The details are printed onto a triple sheet of paper, together with details of the transaction. One sheet of paper is given to the card holder, one sheet is held by the shop and the third sheet is sent to the credit card company.

The credit card company invoices the card holder monthly. Interest is charged if the card holder does not pay all the money outstanding by the time stated on the invoice.

A **standing order** is a method of paying a regular sum of money at a stated time each month, year, or when required. The bank is directed by the account holder to pay a stated amount of money directly from the account into another account.

Direct debit is another system whereby money may be paid by the bank from the account to another account when required. The amount may vary depending on how much is owing at that time.

A **bank statement** is issued by the bank at regular intervals. These may be daily, if the company is a very large one. Monthly is the more usual interval for a small business. A weekly, quarterly or annual statement may be sent as agreed between the bank and the customer.

A **loan** is when money is borrowed, usually for a fixed number of years. Interest is paid at an agreed rate on the money borrowed. Repayment is made monthly. The loan may be short term (2–5 years) or long term (15 or more years).

An **overdraft** is an agreement between the account holder and the bank that more money may be used than is in the account holder's account. Interest is usually charged at a day-to-day rate.

A **creditor** is someone to whom money is owed.

Insolvency is the state where a company or individual is unable to pay their bills. It may be temporary, as when a business requires a loan; or more serious, as when a firm or individual becomes bankrupt.

Bankruptcy is declared when a business faces a total inability to pay its debts. Goods and property may be seized by the Official Receiver and sold to pay the creditors.

Liquidation is the term used when stock is sold off to pay creditors.

Appendix C:
Bookeeping Terminology

A **day cash book** is used to record any cash that is received. The amount of cash should be added up at the end of each day. It should agree with the amount entered in the cash book.

A **cash book** is used to record all money received. This could be in the form of cash, cheques or credit cards. The book should have four columns. The first shows the services given or goods sold, the second shows the total amount of money received. The third shows the amount of VAT that has been paid and the fourth column shows what the actual cost of the service or goods is. Each column should be totalled up each month and cross-checked.

A **petty cash book** is used to record any cash paid out. This is usually used for small purchases such as beverages or cleaning materials.

A **purchase book** is used as a record for anything that is bought. It should have several columns showing to whom the money is paid, the invoice number, the total amount paid, the amount of VAT paid and the total value of the goods without the VAT. Each column should be totalled up each month and agree.

A **wages book** should be kept if any staff are employed. It should show the names of the staff, the total or gross amount being earned, the deductions made for Income Tax and for National Insurance pension contributions. If the staff are part-time, the number of hours that they have worked should be shown.

A **balance sheet** shows a detailed account of all income and expenditure. It is usually drawn up at the end of the financial year.

A **cash flow forecast** is an estimate of the expected income and expenditure of the business over a stated time. This could be a month or a year. It is necessary to draw up a forecast if a loan is required.

A **budget** is an estimate of the expected income for a stated time. By knowing the income it is possible to see if a certain piece of equipment or even extra staff can be afforded.

Depreciation is a term used for the current value of equipment. The value goes down, that is equipment *depreciates* in value each year.

Gross profit is the amount of money received by the business in the course of the year.

Net profit is the amount of profit the business has made after all expenses have been paid.

A **profit and loss account** is a detailed statement showing the income made and expenses paid during a given period of time. It should show which areas of the business are profitable and which areas are making a loss.

Bank reconciliation is a term used for checking the cheque stubs in the cheque book and the paying in book against the bank statement. The cheque number and amount paid out should agree with those in the statement. A note should be made of the cheques that have not been cleared through the account.

VAT (Value Added Tax) is a tax levied on all businesses whose quarterly or annual turnover exceeds a certain amount. This amount is set by the Government and may be altered at any time. It is collected by the Customs and Excise Department. The money is raised by adding a stated amount (17½ per cent at standard rate in 1991) to a wide range of goods and services. In the United Kingdom some goods, such as most food and all children's clothing, are exempt. When the salon turnover reaches the threshold (£35 000) it has to be registered for VAT. All services and goods sold in the salon have to have VAT added to the cost. For example, if a facial treatment is to cost £20, VAT at 17½ per cent will cost an extra £3.50. The total cost to the client will therefore be £23.50. The extra £3.50 is then paid to the Government.

The salon will already have paid VAT on such items as the couch, trolley equipment, bowls, cotton-wool etc. that are required in order to perform e.g. the facial treatment.

There are some advantages to being registered for VAT. The salon has to pay VAT on all items purchased. If the salon is registered for VAT, it can claim the amount paid in VAT back from the Government. For this reason, some businesses register for VAT before reaching the threshold amount. It is also sometimes felt that large businesses may not take as much trouble over a small salon that is not registered for VAT. They may think that the amount of business done with them will be too small to warrant their attention.

If a salon is registered, VAT returns have, by law, to be sent in to the Customs and Excise Department every three months. Failure to do so can lead to a heavy fine or even imprisonment.

Income tax. Everyone earning money is required to pay this tax. The amount depends on a number of factors including marital status, the number of dependents, and the amount of money received from both earned and unearned sources. Some items such as overalls may be set against income tax. If the salon owner is the sole trader all the profit is considered as that one person's income and is therefore taxable. For any staff employed, income tax has to be deducted from the wages before these are handed over. The employer is responsible for paying the employees' income tax. Failure to do so can lead to heavy penalties. Do not hand the money over to the staff to pay their own tax. They may 'forget' to pay it and the salon owner will then have to pay it again to the tax office.

National Insurance is another tax that all employed people are required to pay. The employer is also required to pay part of it. This can be either as weekly contributions – National Insurance stamps can be purchased at the local post office – or by direct debit through the bank.

A bookeeper is a person who may be employed in larger salons to see that all the books are filled in correctly and that the correct salaries are paid etc. Another responsibility may be to see that the cheques are paid to suppliers when due and also to chase up money that may be owing.

An accountant is a most useful person to be able to call upon. They will advise on how to keep the books up-to-date, how to work out the income tax returns, National Insurance contributions and VAT. An accountant can draw up the accounts and agree taxable profits with the Inspector of Taxes. They can advise on what can legally be claimed in tax rebates and often save unnecessary money being paid.

Appendix D: Technical Terminology on Payment of Goods

A **proforma invoice** is an invoice showing which goods have been ordered. The goods are not usually despatched from the company until the money has been received by them. This method of invoicing may be employed when a new customer is applying for goods, when a customer is known to be bad at paying their bills on time or when people have a poor credit rating, when goods are ordered and the cost of them is not known by the customer, or the customer does not have an account with the company.

An **advice note** is an acknowledgement of an order. It may also give the expected date for the goods to be despatched.

A **delivery note** is a list of the items that have been despatched. It is normally written in duplicate. The customer receiving the goods is normally required to sign one copy which is retained by the company. Very often it is used as a verification that the goods have arrived in good order and that the correct goods have been received. The person who receives the goods should sign the note but state that the goods have not been checked. The goods should always be checked against the copy of the delivery note. If any item is damaged or missing, contact the company immediately.

An **invoice** is a list of all the goods ordered and delivered at one time. It should state the cost of each item and also the conditions of sale, and it constitutes a demand for payment. Conditions of sale will vary from company to company. Payment due date may be as little as seven days to as many as thirty days. Each invoice has its own number for record purposes.

A **statement** is a list of all the invoices not paid at a given date. It will contain the invoice number(s) and dates but not the itemised details from the invoice. The statement will usually give details of the date when the money is to be paid. A statement is usually sent out by the company each month.

A **credit note** is often given when goods are returned to the company. This is often given when goods are faulty. A company does not have to give a credit if a salon over-orders and wants to send back the surplus. The amount of credit is usually deducted from the amount of the next invoice.

Useful Addresses

Examining and other Professional Bodies

Confederation of Beauty, Therapy & Cosmetology, 2nd Floor, 34 Imperial Square, Cheltenham, Gloucestershire GL50 1QZ. Tel 0242 570284.

City and Guilds Institute of London, 46 Britannia Street, London WC1 9RG. Tel 071 278 2468.

International Therapy Examination Council, Oakelbrook Mill, Newent, Gloucestershire GL18 1HD. Tel 0531 821875, FAX 0531 822425.

International Federation of Health & Beauty Therapists, PO Box 203, Southampton, Hampshire SO9 7PP. Tel 0703 422695.

National Council for Vocational Qualifications, 222 Euston Road, London NW1 2BZ. Tel 071 387 9898.

Association of Reflexologists, 27 Old Gloucester Street, London WC1N 3XX.

British Reflexology Association, Monks Orchard, Whitbourne, Worcestershire WR6 5RB. Tel 0886 21207.

British Association of Electrologists, 18 Stokes End, Haddenham, Buckinghamshire HP17 8DX. Tel 0844 290721.

Institute of Electrolysis, 251 Seymour Grove, Manchester M16 0DS. Tel 061 881 5306.

International Federation of Aromatherapists, 4 Eastern Road, West Dulwich, London SE21 8HA.

Association of Sun Tanning Organisations, 32 Grayshott Road, London SW11 5TT. Tel 071 228 6077.

Federation of Image Consultants, PO Box 112, Rickmansworth, Hertfordshire WD3 4RE. Tel 0923 897178.

Independent Professional Therapists International (IPTI), 97 London Road, Retford, Nottinghamshire. Tel 0777 700383.

Equipment Suppliers (Training Centres)

Ellisons Ltd, Crondal Road, Exhall, Coventry CV7 9NH. Tel 0203 361619.

Hairdressing & Beauty Equipment Centre, 262 Holloway Road, London N7 6NE. Tel 071 607 7475.

HELP Ltd (Hospital Equipment & Laboratory Products), 2b/3b North Way, Bounds Green Industrial Estate, Bounds Green Road, London N11 2UN. Tel 081 361 9984, FAX 081 361 2815.

Ronald Hagman Ltd, Wendover House, Beaconsfield Road, London N11 3AB. Tel 081 368 3674, FAX 081 361 0372.

George Solly Organisation Ltd, 111 Watlington Street, Reading, Berks RG1 4RQ. Tel 0734 566477, FAX 0734 566318.

Preparations

Hand-made skin-care preparations may be obtained from Ronald Hagman Ltd in salon sizes as well as retail sizes. A number of beauty and therapy products are also available. These include over 70 pure essential oils for professional blending as well as essential oils pre-blended with vitoleum, ready for aromatherapeutic uses. Formulation and 'own salon label' can also be supplied.

J.M.R. Paramedical Products, 17 Rossett Holt Close, Harrogate HG2 9AD. Tel 0423 505707.

House of Neroli at Oakelbrook Mill, Newent, Gloucestershire GL18 1HD. Tel 0531 821875, FAX 0531 822425.

Insurance

Hairdressers Insurance, Rockwood House, 9–17 Perrymount Road, Haywards Heath, West Sussex RH16 1TA. Tel 0444 458144. Available to all members of the Association of Beauty, Therapy and Cosmeticology.

Trade Journals

Health and Beauty Salon, Quadrant House, The Quadrant, Sutton, Surrey SM2 5AS. Tel 081 661 3500.

Les Nouvelles Estatiques, 7 avenue Stèphane-Mallarmè, 75017 Paris, FRANCE.

Index

205